HUMAN
HEALTHCARE

Patterns of Hope for a
System under Strain

Dr Margaret Hannah

Published by:
Triarchy Press
Station Offices
Axminster
Devon
EX13 5PF
United Kingdom

+44 (0)1297 631456
info@triarchypress.net
www.triarchypress.net

© International Futures Forum, 2014

A catalogue record for this book is available from the British Library.

ISBN: 978-1-909470-44-6

Artwork by Jennifer Williams

Contents

Introduction 1

PART 1: THE CONTEMPORARY CHALLENGE

CHAPTER 1
The House that Modern Medicine Built 9

CHAPTER 2
Overweight and Overwhelmed 20

CHAPTER 3
Costing an Arm and a Leg 36

PART 2: THE RESPONSE

CHAPTER 4
The Brakes are Failing 49

CHAPTER 5
Regulation, Inspection and
the Fight Against Error 59

CHAPTER 6
RCTs: A Self-Limiting Improvement Methodology 69

PART 3: ANOTHER WAY IS POSSIBLE

CHAPTER 7
The Patterning of Hope 81

CHAPTER 8
Designing for Transition 110

CHAPTER 9
Creating the Future 118

End Notes 137

Introduction

"Humankind has managed to get people to the moon, created devices which connect us with others anywhere in the world, and made 640 tonnes of metal fly through the air, so why can't we find a sustainable model for healthcare?"
Anoop Maini, *The Guardian*, 12 August 2013

Healthcare systems across the developed world are under strain. Whether their funding is public, private or hybrid, they all face a potentially crippling combination of insatiable demand and rising costs of supply.

There has for a long time been a touching faith, not supported by the evidence, that some combination of smart reorganisation, financial innovation to shift costs and incentives, rigorously disciplined efficiency plus better health education for the public will be enough to see us through. That confidence is now beginning to crack – not least as recent attempts to ratchet down costs in the wake of the financial crisis have offered only temporary relief and healthcare spending across the OECD countries starts to rise again.

This should come as no surprise. A survey in 2005 by Healthcast 2020, PricewaterhouseCoopers' health research institute, revealed that most healthcare executives in the developed world expected healthcare costs to increase to 2020 at a higher rate than in the past. That was a reflection based on the experience of their professional lives, and of my own. Yet the same report, in a later chapter on 'The Unsustainability of Global Health Systems', acknowledged the truth that these trends cannot possibly continue indefinitely.

Similarly in my own organisation, the UK National Health Service, there is a growing sense of urgency about the need for radical change in order to keep the system going. Seventy percent of NHS leaders recently surveyed are not confident we can do so with the limited playbook of healthcare reform options we have been drawing on for decades.

I share that view — which is why I wrote this book. It falls into three parts: a deep diagnosis of the problem, a review of the inadequacy of the current menu of technical remedies, and a final section offering the foundations for a more hopeful approach that draws on the underlying strengths of both professionals and patients.

The first part of this book explores why healthcare costs in the modern world have become an ever-increasing proportion of economic activity. This is not the result of poor policy or failures of efficiency (even if both can be improved). It is a consequence rather of an underlying and largely invisible set of beliefs which underpin the structures and behaviours of modern healthcare.

For over two centuries medicine has drawn from and contributed to a mechanistic worldview that has tended to see the body as a machine and medicine as an episodic service of fix and repair. This has been very successful in many different ways, but it has also fed a distinctive pattern of growth based on technical capacity. Can't we make the machine go faster? Make it more efficient? Enhance it to make it last forever? As former President of the Royal College of General Practitioners, Iona Heath, puts it, medicine is being pressed to provide "technical solutions to existential problems".

Healthcare systems built on this view of the world have struggled to adapt and respond to today's changing patterns of disease. Patients treated in hospital today are much older than their counterparts even a generation ago, they have chronic diseases, they are more in need of care than cure and often lack close family and friends to help them recover at home. We are also confronted by the rise in conditions that are more obviously the result of complex social factors rather than simply the physiology of the individual. Obesity, addiction and inequalities in health have been on the rise since the early 1980s. For the first time ever in peacetime we are now facing the prospect of a generation of parents outliving their children.

Meanwhile the healthcare systems we designed for another age are everywhere subject to 'healthcare inflation'. Part of this is driven by medical technology. As techniques expand, experience with them deepens and their safety is more assured, they become available for more people. It is not uncommon for frail 90-year-olds to have hip replacement surgery, for example. At the same time commercial interests encourage greater use of certain drugs, diagnostics and products. Doctors alter the thresholds for prescribing drugs on the basis of research funded for the most part by drug companies. In the UK general practitioners are subject to a contract which includes financial incentives for prescribing certain drugs and offering specific screening tests. Despite our best efforts to contain it, healthcare inflation now seems locked into the present system.

The second part of the book reviews the range of responses we have developed to date to tackle this problematic combination of decreasing effectiveness in the face of new patterns of disease and continuing cost pressures eroding financial viability.

There is a range of supply side interventions – reducing costs, improving efficiency, consolidating services. There are attempts to limit demand – through health improvement, treatment thresholds, varieties of rationing. There is the whole burgeoning apparatus of inspection, regulation and quality control designed to get the best out of a system already under strain. And running through it all is a research and innovation philosophy (isolate a single element and see whether we can improve it) evidently at odds with the reality of a complex human social system. If these are the brakes on a system heading towards the cliff edge, we must conclude that they are failing.

What these approaches miss, consistent with a dominant view of the human as machine, are the infinite resources that feed life and how to tap into them. The third part of the book describes examples of healthcare systems I have encountered that are founded on a very different set of premises. That health is a product of healthy relationships, a quality of life held in common. That nobody can be healthy alone. That given the right conditions health is contagious and can spread like an infectious disease. And that who we are being as healthcare professionals is as important as what we are doing. These insights have provided the basis for my own evolving practice in recent years. They suggest to me a future patterning of hope.

Chapter 7 describes a healthcare system based on these insights and operating at scale – the 'Nuka' model of care in Alaska, which I have had the privilege to visit and learn from on a number of occasions. 'Nuka' is an Alaskan Native word for a strong and extensive living structure. Healthcare in this system is based on reconnecting people into this web of life. No less an authority than Don Berwick, a former health adviser to President Obama and a founder of the highly respected Institute for Healthcare Improvement, has declared that Nuka "is probably the leading example of healthcare redesign in the world. US healthcare suffers from high costs and low quality. This system has reversed that: the quality of care is the highest I have seen anywhere in the world, and the costs are highly sustainable. It's extraordinary. It is surely leading healthcare to its new and proper destination."

Having explored some of the features of this radically effective and affordable system of healthcare we can start to recognise aspects of this new pattern already occurring at small scale elsewhere, including around the UK. The success of these so far isolated experiments in enacting a new model encourages us to do more and makes it possible to imagine a radical renewal within the NHS such that it can provide once again a health system which is universal, free at the point of delivery and meeting contemporary patterns of illness as part of an integrated approach that sustains healthy, fulfilled lives at a fraction of the current cost.

The final chapters describe how this might be achieved. The transition already under way can be supported by a smarter policy landscape designed to encourage it. And practitioners at all levels in the system can start to grow – or in most cases to rediscover – this new culture of healthcare within their current practice.

None of this could have been written without the support of International Futures Forum. For over a decade IFF has been developing the conceptual and the practical tools to help people trying to make a difference in the world in the face of all that stands in the way of making a difference. The challenges facing healthcare systems have their parallels in many other modern institutions – education, criminal justice, banking, the media. IFF is clear that the crisis is cultural not technical, and that the level of thinking that led us into it is not going to be enough to get us out.

The book has been written for the general reader, but has particular messages for practitioners, policy makers and thought leaders in the field of healthcare. It is not intended to offer a grand solution to what is a complex web of interacting challenges, but rather to give legitimacy and authority to a new perspective that opens up largely unexplored territory in the debate about the future of healthcare in the UK and elsewhere around the world.

What lies ahead is not just an assimilation of this new thinking but a challenge for all of us to re-examine the assumptions that underpin our own practice. At present, whether as patients or professionals, we sit anxiously in the surgery while experts reveal the results of yet another battery of tests that show the healthcare system is in crisis. They offer a bewildering array of more or less aggressive technical interventions designed to hold the crisis at bay. Yet we sense the consultation needs to go deeper than that. We know the mechanistic mindset is now offering diminishing returns. We need to find a place again in the conversation for hope, meaning, purpose – and for Nuka.

This is a cultural transition. Former California State Senator John Vasconcellos suggests that what we therefore face is a double task. We must become "hospice workers for the dying culture and midwives for the new". In my experience the hospice work is the more difficult part of this equation. Existing patterns of power, competence and authority are reluctant to make space for other ways of practising – however effective the results. At best, we can expect scepticism and resistance; at worst, active suppression.

But the results will speak for themselves. If there is one lesson from this book and from my own experience in recent years it is that human systems have the power to transform themselves and nothing short of a complete transformation will be enough to address the greatest health crisis of our times. I hope, dear reader, you will take courage from these tales of cultural change already happening in healthcare and be ready to play your part in co-creating its future.

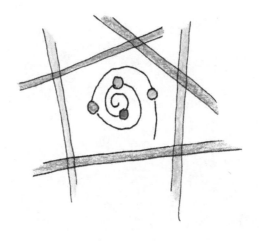

PART 1:

THE CONTEMPORARY CHALLENGE

CHAPTER 1

The House that Modern Medicine Built

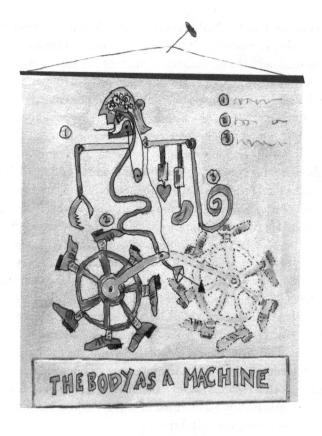

THE BODY AS A MACHINE

*"Each generation must examine and think through again, from
its own distinct vantage point, the ideas that have shaped its
understanding of the world."*
Richard Tarnas, *The Passion of the Western Mind*, 1991

Modern medicine has built its success on a deep understanding
of the body as a machine. It is this understanding that has
determined both the fundamental nature of the encounter
between doctor and patient and the vast infrastructure of
complex healthcare systems that has grown up to serve it. It
is beguilingly simple: take a history from the sick person, seek
out specific details which cover a range of pre-existing disease
states, physically examine the body (or mentally examine the
mind), come to a conclusion about what is wrong and fix it. With
advances in drug and surgical treatments in the last century,
especially for infections and traumatic injuries as well as problems
with worn-out parts, this approach has been hugely successful,
and has transformed the odds of us all living to a ripe old age.

This progress has been hard won. Understanding the body as
a machine required a radical breakthrough in thinking centuries
ago, derived from an early interest in anatomy. Whilst this can
be traced to ancient Egypt and Greece, the modern objective
exploration of the body began in earnest in the 16th and 17th
centuries. The early pioneers of modern medicine used dissection
of the human body as a fundamental source of knowledge.
Vesalius is often regarded as its founder although we now know
that Leonardo da Vinci undertook many dissections but did not
publish his drawings in his lifetime.

In his treatise *De humani corporis fabrica* (1543) Vesalius
challenged the previous orthodoxy based on Galen's work in
the 2nd century – that our health is the result of an imbalance in
humours (black and yellow bile, blood and phlegm). Vesalius's
book, in seven volumes, was lavishly illustrated with detailed
diagrams of the key structures of the human body – heart, lungs,

liver, gut, arteries, veins, bones and muscle. As David Armstrong
has described, in this way the body became legible through a new
language of structure and description, based on the objective
evidence of human dissection[1].

Early modern doctors learned to read the body through
anatomical eyes and, in doing so, were starting to see the body
as object rather than subject, to 'objectify' their gaze. This shift
created a distance between the experience of inhabiting the body
and its external description. The first is unique to every person,
connecting to their family, community and life in its widest
sense. The latter is de-contextualised, focusing on structures
and function at the same time, opening up the possibility of new
understandings about how the body works. Thus William Harvey
was able to describe the circulation of the blood for the first time
in 1628, not just describing the structure of arteries and veins
but likening the flow of blood through the heart to that of liquid
through a mechanical pump. This discovery had the interesting
corollary of making the King's heart no different from those of
his subjects. Some argue this shift in worldview made it easier for
the rise of democracy and an end to the divine right of Kings[2].

In time, doctors came to identify this anatomical, mechanical
map of the body as the actual territory rather than just one of
many possible representations. Similarly, doctors began to cluster
symptoms and signs in the patients who came to them and labeled
them as 'diseases', giving them specific names.

In order to develop this systematic knowledge and
understanding of medicine, students started to learn from
lectures and textbooks, dissection of corpses, and the hands-
on examination of patients who were being treated in teaching
hospitals. These establishments became big, powerful
institutions, attracting the best medical men (it was all men
for over a century) to teach in them. Doctors in turn gained
reputations, which allowed them to charge high fees for their
private practice.

The training of doctors along these lines socialised them into seeing illness and suffering in a particular way and created a distance between them and the lived experience of their patients. This led to the emergence of what Michel Foucault described as the "clinical gaze"[3]. It means seeing people as bundles of symptoms or data or diagnoses rather than as themselves. The clinical gaze might be detected in the kind of conversation that can happen between doctors when they refer to a sick person on a ward as "the lymphoma in the corner". I found myself caught up in this world when I was practising hospital medicine. Even the persistence of the word 'patient' for a person experiencing illness is a manifestation of the passivity of the role compared with the active role of diagnosis and treatment by the doctor.

The clinical gaze is not just about the way doctors view patients. It represents a whole worldview which defines roles, relationships, what knowledge is taken seriously, and what is not, how power is exercised and how healthcare is organised. The process is sub-conscious, not a conspiracy, but it leads to a clear demarcation of roles in modern healthcare.

Medical knowledge and skill are highly prized and protected as a scare resource and doctors remain well-paid professionals. Nurses have attempted to emulate that success by becoming a graduate–level entry profession, codifying their knowledge and skills in the same way. Other healthcare professionals have followed suit, each group with its own training and professional organisation.

With advances in psychology and sociology in the 1960s and 1970s, this bio-mechanical model of disease was criticised for failing to take into account the wider circumstances in people's lives, which have both an impact on the development of disease and implications for how it might be treated. Most medical schools today teach the 'bio-psycho-social' model of disease, which incorporates psychological and social influences when making a diagnosis.

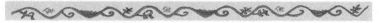

However, despite these adjustments, doctors still locate the pathology of disease in individual patients and remedies still focus on physical or behavioural levels of intervention. Clearly, psychiatry is different – recognising that a person with a disordered mind needs psychological and social support often over many years. However, even here, the prevailing view is that psychiatric disorders such as schizophrenia and bi-polar disorder are largely the consequence of chemical imbalances in the brain.

Production-line healthcare

Today's medicine is largely practised within multi-disciplinary teams comprising many different professionals. In theory this opens up the opportunity for a more integrated view of disease and treatment. For example, a stroke unit may have doctors, nurses, physiotherapists, speech and language therapists, occupational therapists and psychologists working together for the optimal treatment of people who have had strokes. However, the knowledge and skills of each professional group do not fundamentally change the clinical gaze — they each simply fill in further detail. The disease is still located in the individual and the treatment is largely co-ordinated around them.

Because so many professional perspectives are needed to treat health problems today many conditions now have to be managed through specific 'care pathways', akin to production lines in manufacturing. Once someone is admitted with a stroke, for example, they receive input from a variety of different professionals at specified times in the course of their treatment and recovery. This pattern of care has been called 'integrated', but in reality it is additive. Each professional plays their part in a highly co-ordinated, structured and essentially mechanical way, adding layers of expertise into the treatment programme.

With this understanding of how clinical knowledge and practice has built up over the years, it becomes clear why healthcare inflation persists in spite of overall improvements in health in the last fifty years. As the field of knowledge expands and includes more disciplines, more niches within the healthcare system become occupied. These different disciplines need to come together to provide care and treatment for individual patients, so the process becomes more complicated and further resources are needed for co-ordination.

The result of all this activity has been incremental improvement in outcomes of healthcare through the accumulation of marginal gains. In areas of excellence, the precision and co-ordination of activity is impressive. Like mechanics attending a Formula-one racing car in a pit-stop, every member of the team is focused on their part of the task: replacing worn parts, refilling fuel and lubricants, checking all systems are functioning as expected and doing so at break-neck speed to get the car back out on the track.

But the process has limits. Shaving further seconds off the time taken to drive round the circuit requires progressively more effort. This is the law of diminishing returns and is quite evident in healthcare today. In the UK the health budget almost doubled between 2000 and 2010 but the improvement in outcomes was modest. Waiting times were reduced and public satisfaction rose, but to continue to improve at this rate would require an exponential growth in spending with ever decreasing gains for the level of additional investment.

The Birth of the Clinic

Foucault has described how the organisation of healthcare and disease categorisation went hand in hand with the birth of the clinic in the 19th century. This process has shaped the power dynamics and design of healthcare settings ever since.

When hospitals were first created they were very much for the poor. If you were rich the doctor would come to see you at home. Now, the size of specialist teams and equipment, laboratories and the need for sterile environments mean that hospitals have

grown in size and complexity and because of economies of scale are often located far from people's homes. Furthermore, the spatial separation of the patient from his or her home setting removes complex influences on the clinical picture presented to the doctor. It has the effect of negating personal and relational aspects of the causes and effects of the illness, whilst enhancing the disease-focused attention of the clinical gaze. Distancing the patient's personal circumstances from the frame privileges one form of knowledge over another and shifts the balance of power in healthcare systems from the person seeking help to the supplier.

The extent to which we have lock-in to this model is exemplified by the design of a modern hospital where the spatial segregation is remarkable. There are departments for different parts (ophthalmology) and systems of the body (neurology), different types of diagnostic method (xray, labs) and different types of therapy (OT, physio). The biggest spatial separation lies between illnesses that affect mainly the mind (psychiatry) and those that affect mainly the body. In many cases, people are treated in separate hospitals if they are diagnosed with both a physical and a mental illness.

These observations illustrate the cumulative effect of one perspective — the clinical gaze — on the design of healthcare. Even the word 'clinical' has gained a somewhat sinister connotation, meaning an approach that is cold and calculating whilst being highly precise. Similarly the term 'surgical strike' denotes a form of precision bombardment. Such language reflects the remoteness of this way of thinking from the lay-person and suggests a shadow side to gleaming wards and white coats. The science of anatomy itself is predicated on dissecting a dead body. Learning the physical location of organs and tissues in the body through dissection requires a psychological split for young medical students, much of which is compensated for by black humour.

This separation of the observer from the observed creates a distance between clinical staff and patients. There are understandable psychological reasons for this, mostly associated with anxiety — about death, sickness, pain and loss of control of bodily functions[4]. However, there are consequences, most notably in the fragmentation of the patient experience. Whilst different clinicians determine the best way to organise healthcare around their own specialisms, each creating a niche for developing expertise, patients feel lost and alienated. Careful attention to 'customer care' can alter this experience but fundamentally modern healthcare is provider-driven rather than designed around the needs of the people seeking help.

As noted above, for all the talk of broadening beyond a 'bio-medical model' to embrace psychological and social factors, the clinical gaze still tends to locate illness in individuals. This ignores a great deal of the complexity in the way that illness actually manifests in people's lives. A cranial CT scan, for example, will not help to find the cause of a person's headache if they are stressed by their partner's infidelities, financial worries or are being bullied at work. Focusing on lowering individual risk factors such as cholesterol or high blood pressure is unlikely to be effective in preventing heart disease if someone continues to be stressed because of poverty, poor working conditions or family problems. Screening tests, even if they are worthwhile (which is highly marginal in some cases), are unlikely to be taken up by busy working mums with children and ageing parents to worry about.

The Demand for Certainty

It is in the nature of the clinical gaze to seek consistency, reliability, predictability and certainty. In reality, making a diagnosis is much more hazy than either doctors or the public like to think. Despite the emphasis on precision and clarity, results from medical investigations can be interpreted very differently in

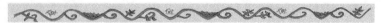

practice. Studies have shown that when pathologists review each other's slides they can reach different views on whether a tissue biopsy is cancerous or not[5]. When a laboratory reports blood chemistry results, these results provide a reference range within which the majority of people lie, yet there may be results outside this range which are not the result of underlying pathology. The results may just be normal for that particular person at the time the sample was taken, or the way the sample was taken and processed may not have been satisfactory. Likewise, imaging techniques may reveal what appears to be a cancerous growth which turns out to be benign. Whatever measuring methods are used, they carry a level of uncertainty.

People want clear answers to the questions, "What's wrong with me?" or "Is it serious?". Yet often diagnosis is not clear cut. Doctors and their patients have to balance uncertainty in diagnosis with the risks of continuing down an investigative route. Doctors have different thresholds for tolerating this uncertainty. Generally, more experienced clinicians and those working in general practice are more able to bear this uncertainty when compared with junior hospital doctors who are more likely to order tests, make referrals to other specialities and generate higher costs.

The clinical gaze also feeds a culture that drives towards cure seemingly at any cost. This seems justifiable when we are 'fighting for our lives'. The stakes can be high. Considering the history of advances in medicine, the use of military language to describe our efforts to 'combat' disease should not come as a surprise. Ambulance services began in the First World War, when it became clear that survival rates from injury were better if soldiers were treated quickly by skilled surgeons a little way back from the frontline. Plastic surgery developed as a speciality through dealing with disfigurement from blasts and gunshot wounds. Even today new techniques such as early, massive blood transfusions are improving the survival rates of soldiers injured in Iraq and Afghanistan.

There is no debate: where acute and possibly fatal conditions arise, modern medicine has no rival and heroic, invasive methods have proved invaluable. But for the most part modern medicine is not dealing with battlefield situations. The chronic, relapsing burden of disease in the 21st century is unlikely to be tackled effectively through biomechanical thinking and military-style delivery systems.

The idea that we are up against an enemy when 'fighting' disease also reflects the era when bacteria were discovered to be the cause of many common conditions and the use of antiseptic methods became established as a means of avoiding infection. Such thinking persists in advertisements today for bathroom cleaning agents, which are represented as the 'frontline' in keeping the house free of germs. Frequently drugs and other treatments are designed to be combatants against disease. We have long lists of 'antis': anti-biotics, anti-histamines, anti-inflammatories, anti-tumour drugs.

The idea of battling disease has become ingrained, but it is not clear who is the combatant. Christopher Hitchens was asked about his "battle against cancer" before he died, but was clearly caught by how inappropriate the metaphor felt in practice: "What I feel is that this [the cancer] is making war on me. I'm the one being battled, and it has the advantage — it's taken the initiative. When I go to the clinic next and sit with a tube in my arm and watch the poison go in, I'm in an attitude of abject passivity. It doesn't feel like fighting at all; it just feels like submitting."

Whilst illness and suffering is a human struggle, requiring strength and fortitude to pull through, using a military metaphor like the 'war against cancer' closes down many other options for addressing the health challenges we face in the 21st century[6]. It is interesting to note that the military mindset itself is moving to a much more nuanced view of contemporary warfare in an age of low-level conflict and local insurgency. So, sadly, we are more likely to hear military generals discussing a strategy to win the hearts and minds of the populace while our surgeons and consultants still dream of winning the battle against disease through superior forces and better kit.

ℰ Reflection

If we are to engage in an honest debate about the future of healthcare systems we need to acknowledge the limits of mechanistic thinking and the fundamental assumptions underpinning the clinical gaze. They have worked wonders in their day and will continue to play their part in the future but cannot any longer remain the dominant belief system to the exclusion of all others. They cannot underpin a different model of healthcare which offers real hope for progress in the face of a new pattern of disease, coupled with long-term financial sustainability. It is to these twin challenges that we now turn.

CHAPTER 2

Overweight and Overwhelmed

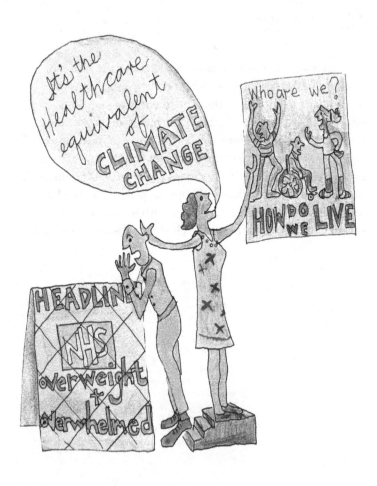

"I am not a mechanism, an assembly of various sections.
And it is not because the mechanism is working wrongly, that
I am ill."

D H Lawrence, "Healing"

We have seen how the practice of medicine has developed empirically, understanding the body as a machine and diseases as identifiable and discrete with analytically discernable symptoms and readily available technical treatments. But today's pattern of disease is much more complex than this — and challenges us to develop more effective approaches.

Back in the 1940s when the NHS was established, the main reasons for admission to hospital were acute infections, accidents and the need for surgery. Today we see a greater number of cases of chronic disease, sometimes existing together as 'multiple morbidity', generated or exacerbated by underlying problems such as obesity, depression, anxiety, dementia, smoking, alcohol and drug dependency. These are complex conditions for which a mechanistic response will not work. Complex problems present a different kind of challenge compared with complicated ones[7]. To use an analogy: a car engine is complicated but any well-trained mechanic can isolate a fault and remedy it. In contrast, the impact of the car on society is complex — unpredictable, multi-faceted and disruptive.

Complex problems need to be addressed in their entirety, not piece-by-piece. They cannot be 'solved' or controlled, but we can learn to work with them[8]. For example, with complex patterns of disease it is difficult for a person to know exactly when they are unwell: often they feel a general sense of malaise, of not being up to par, with non-specific symptoms and many ups and downs. For the doctor, unlike for traumatic injury or acute infection, the best course of treatment is uncertain and even more so if a patient has more than one chronic condition. A further question hangs over recovery: with chronic health problems, it might not be possible to return to your previous life.

This chapter highlights some of the more obvious evidence of the changing pattern of disease — the rise in obesity, stress, mental health problems, addictions and so on — and also society-wide effects of inequality, austerity and demographic change. It concludes with the observation that at root this changing pattern is *cultural:* it is changes in the culture, in the way we live our lives, that underlie the new pattern of disease, and addressing the effects of these changes lies way beyond the reach of the biomechanical model.

Overweight

There is widespread recognition that obesity is a risk factor for developing many common diseases such as diabetes, heart and liver disease and some cancers. But the scale is perhaps less well understood. We are in the midst of a pandemic of obesity-related ill health.

In England alone in the five years from 2006 to 2011 the number of people diagnosed with diabetes increased by 25%, from 1.9 million to 2.5 million[9]. About 80% of these people are overweight and the rise in Type 2 diabetes, which makes up most of this increase, is in line with the rise of obesity in society. Diabetes is now the biggest single cause of amputation, stroke, blindness and end-stage kidney failure in the UK.

Obesity also leads to complications following childbirth and adds risks when giving anaesthetics. It increases the likelihood of complications following surgery and slows down the speed of recovery from illness. Even the basic infrastructure of hospitals and clinics has had to adapt to the rise in obesity, with wider trolleys, more powerful hoists, bigger beds and chairs, and specialist mattresses to prevent bed sores.

Healthcare has neither prevented obesity nor found a way to reverse the rising trend in people who need to reduce their

weight. Some 35% of the adult population in the US is now obese, compared with 15% thirty-five years ago. The figure for the UK is over 25%. Weight gain is insidious. In Scotland, the population is averaging a one kilogram increase per person per year. If you assume obesity is a consequence of an imbalance between calories in and calories expended, this is the equivalent of no more than an extra two biscuits per day. It does not take much to sustain a rising trend in obesity. There is a view that the form in which calories are taken may also play a part in encouraging weight gain, but even this does not explain why obesity has become such a major health issue across the globe.

A UK Government Foresight Report in 2007 described a vast number of inter-connecting factors which combine to generate the changing shape and size of people's waistlines[10]. This is a complex phenomenon, not a complicated one, and is intimately tied to the way we lead our lives in the modern world. The report concluded that we live in an "obesogenic society" and it will require a major culture shift to change this.

Meanwhile, healthcare systems around the world are responding to the rising trend in obesity-related illness with last-ditch methods. Bariatric surgery (e.g. gastric banding or gastric bypassing) offers the only hope for some people of avoiding early death. But the operation is not without its difficulties. 1% of people die following surgery and 10% have serious complications. People need to change their dietary habits for life and doctors have to monitor them closely to make sure they do not run into long-term problems. For many others, weight management programmes have been of limited success. At best, they delay further weight gain rather than achieve substantial and sustainable weight loss. Health education messages have not been successful either. Telling people to eat less and exercise more has been the mantra for several decades and yet obesity in the adult population is now at unprecedented levels.

In reality, modern healthcare methods have no lasting and effective solution to the rising trend in obesity. Instead we face

a huge burden of morbidity and a pressure on costs without any
clear strategies for stemming the tide.

Overwhelmed

Mental health problems are now responsible for a bigger share
of spend in health systems than heart disease or cancer. These
problems often co-exist with physical health problems, yet
services are usually separated, not just into different departments
within hospitals, but into separate hospitals. Depression alone is
associated with many other illnesses and problems including heart
disease, alcohol dependency, self-harm and suicide. People who
are depressed are more likely to succumb to infection and take
longer to recover. At the same time, many people experiencing
chronic disease get depressed. A vicious cycle is created whereby
more people survive with chronic disease but become depressed
as the disease drags on. The depression makes people vulnerable
to more illness and more depression. These patterns of disease-
on-disease are not uncommon and lead to multiple visits to
doctors for tests and treatments. The main burden for this extra
work is falling on general practice.

Like obesity, the rising rates of mental health problems such
as depression, anxiety, addictions, self-harm and suicide are a
reflection of the lives we lead. Early childhood events such as
neglect, abuse, bereavement or having a parent with mental
illness all contribute to risk as do social deprivations such as
unemployment, low income and poor housing. Loneliness,
poor quality human relationships, lack of belonging, and loss of
meaning and purpose can cause depression but can also be the
effects of the condition, generating a negative cycle. This is partly
why depression can be such a debilitating and recurring problem
in people's lives. People who have struggled to have trusting and
life-enhancing relationships are more likely to become depressed
and feel unworthy. People who are depressed because they feel

unworthy are less likely to trust others or accept love when they are offered it.

The healthcare system's response to mental health problems has been mainly drug treatment and a limited range of talking therapies. Drugs may have been important in reducing the risk of suicide in severely depressed people. However, many people with depression have mild to moderate illness and in those cases the impact of drug treatment is more limited.

In England in 2009 there were 40 million prescriptions for anti-depressant drugs such as Prozac. This is four times higher than the level in 1991. This steep rise is partly because doctors are diagnosing and treating depression more, but also because they prescribe anti-depressants for a year to eighteen months whereas previously they were given for shorter courses of three or four months only. Talking therapies, such as cognitive behavioural therapy, have increased in popularity but in the NHS are usually offered in tightly scheduled programmes of six to eight sessions - partly because the scientific evidence is supportive of short courses, but also because the cost of longer courses would be prohibitive.

Stress and inequality

Chronic stress causes many health problems, not just anxiety and depression. It is one of the main factors contributing to patterns of health inequality observed in modern society. Where there is a big difference in income and wealth between the least and most affluent, premature death from heart disease and cancer show a steep gradient. This gradient is repeated across a wide range of conditions, including depression, alcohol and drug-related problems, violence, accidents and maternal and infant mortality. In the UK income inequalities widened markedly during the 1980s and 1990s and have persisted despite efforts at progressive tax and welfare policies by the Blair/Brown governments[11].

Wilkinson and Pickett have shown that it is not only the health of the poorest sections that fares so badly in unequal societies - the health and wellbeing of the whole population suffers[12]. Michael Marmot has called the underlying stress of inequality "status syndrome"[13]. He has described at the biological level how this interferes with our metabolism, affecting the immune system, blood pressure and insulin sensitivity. The chronic stress of living on a low income in the face of others who don't have to worry about money in effect accelerates the process of ageing. Premature deaths from cancer and heart disease are often the end result.

Healthcare systems have been slow to respond to widening health inequalities. Effort is focused on ensuring hospitals and clinics are compliant with legislation regarding equality and diversity, for example ensuring disabled access to buildings, encouraging recruitment from minority groups and raising awareness in the workforce of their legal duties. But pay differentials in healthcare organisations are widening. In 1999, chief executives of NHS organisations were paid three and a half times as much as nurses on average. Ten years later that figure had risen to five times[14].

Arguably, certain healthcare activities have themselves widened health inequalities. For example, health education messages to stop smoking and eat a healthy diet have been adopted more quickly by affluent people. Smoking is largely confined to poor people in the UK today. If you are not worried about the price of food, it is easier to eat a healthy diet. People on low incomes are more likely to delay seeking medical attention when they are ill. Conversely, better-educated and more affluent people navigate their way around the healthcare system more successfully.

Furthermore, many doctors choose to work in more comfortable circumstances. Julian Tudor Hart proposed the 'inverse care law' which observes that health facilities tend to be

located in more affluent areas, where less healthcare is needed[15]. In the US this is particularly marked and has a paradoxical effect: where there are facilities there is more healthcare regardless of whether or not it is warranted[16]. For example, in cities where there are a lot of hospitals undertaking coronary artery stent operations, more people have the operation. The provision of the service is a higher predictor of being treated than the level of need in the population, and treatment is available on the basis of an ability to pay.

An age of austerity

Since the 2008 financial crash and economic recession, financial worries, insecure employment, cuts in welfare benefits along with rising costs of food, fuel and other basics have seen increasing levels of stress in the population with subsequent damage to health. Suicide rates in men in England aged 45 to 59 have risen significantly since 2007[17]. In Greece, Spain and Ireland too, mental health problems are escalating.

Welfare systems, which historically have offset the worst aspects of inequality, are being cut back as governments attempt to deal with their structural deficits. These austerity measures are increasing the income gap between the richest and poorest, reducing staffing levels in healthcare and increasing demand. In Greece wages for doctors and nurses have been slashed, needle exchange schemes abandoned (leading to more HIV infection in IV drug users) and there is a resurgence of infectious diseases as sanitation and control measures, such as mosquito spraying programmes, are cut back. The health impact has been worse than researchers predicted. Malaria is now circulating in Greece after the country had been clear of the infection for 40 years[18]. Suicide and murder rates have increased by 23% and 28% respectively between 2007 and 2009[19]. In the USA deaths from suicide now exceed those from car accidents. Whilst the latter have fallen 25% over ten years to 2010, suicides have gone up by 30% in the same period[20].

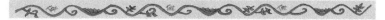

Other austerity measures include changing welfare rules. Many people with disabilities in the UK have to demonstrate again and again that they are unable to work for a living before they can claim benefits. These assessments can feel highly stressful for the disabled person. On the one hand people want to make the best of what they can do and don't want to talk themselves down. On the other hand they need to be honest about their limitations if they are to obtain the payments to which they are entitled. Many disabled people, particularly those with mental health problems, become agitated and distressed as their assessment appointment comes close. Should they need to appeal against a decision, this stress can last for months. All of this adds up to a higher likelihood of disabled people becoming ill and needing medical attention.

Addictions

Just like obesity and mental health problems, the rise in addictions is a consequence of the way we lead our lives. Addictions are not limited to drug and alcohol dependency, but can include tobacco, sex, gambling, work, pornography, body-building, TV watching and internet browsing. These addictions can lead to a variety of health problems such as chest infections, lung cancer, sexually-transmitted infections, stress and burn-out, sleep problems, inappropriate use of anabolic steroids and poor work performance.

The healthcare response to addiction has been mixed. Since the early 1980s there has been significant success in reducing the harm caused by sharing needles by providing needle exchange schemes for heroin users. In addition, there appear to be signs that the tide of heroin abuse is turning, with fewer young people taking up the habit. Investment in detoxification, relapse prevention and rehabilitation services appears to be paying off where drug addiction is concerned, with a greater proportion of people now leaving rehab to find new pathways in their lives and not coming back[21].

However, the picture is less impressive for the far greater number of people with alcohol dependency. Generally speaking specialist alcohol services are in short supply — on average only one in twenty people in England needing this level of support for an alcohol problem is offered it[22]. Admissions to hospital due to alcohol in England are now at record levels[23]. Alcohol-related liver disease is the leading cause of cirrhosis and demand for liver transplants. Deaths from alcohol-related problems increased dramatically in the 1990s and 2000s, reaching a plateau in 2009 in England although now showing a slight decline.

Childhood trauma

Psychiatrists have long known about a link between childhood experience and adult mental health problems, including depression, self-harm, addictions, suicide and violence. What is less well known is that adverse events can have physical health effects too. The effects of experiences of domestic violence, abuse or neglect are cumulative. The more adverse events in childhood, the more likely a person is to develop ischaemic heart disease, cancer, chronic obstructive lung disease, bone fractures and liver disease[24].

These findings were first published in 1998 but their impact on medical practice has been negligible. Although it is routine for paediatricians and child psychiatrists to ask about and look for evidence of abuse, very few doctors who look after adults ask about what happened in childhood as part of their enquiry. This has potentially harmful consequences. Consider vaginal or anal examinations, looking down the throat for signs of infection, dental treatment and smear tests. They can all act as triggers for flashbacks in someone who has been sexually abused as a child. Healthcare is not just failing to adapt to the changing patterns of disease, it may be putting off the very people who need its care the most.

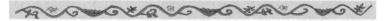

Demographic change

Over the last century, largely through better living and working
conditions, better nutrition and better maternal and child health,
life expectancy has increased. People are living longer, but often
with chronic disease. This is in some part attributable to modern
medicine, which has converted previously fatal conditions into
chronic ones. In addition, the risk of developing diseases such as
heart disease, stroke, cancer, arthritis and diabetes increases with
age. There are also conditions, associated with ageing itself, such
as frailty and dementia, which are having a significant impact on
healthcare systems. As a result of these factors nearly half of all
hospital in-patients are over the age of 60. A quarter are aged
over 75.

One of the reasons for high levels of in-patient bed use by
older people is the time it takes for rehabilitation from illness.
If a frail older person falls down at home with no-one there
to help get them up, in many cases they are taken to hospital.
Simply entering a different environment can be very upsetting
for someone with dementia, sight- or hearing- loss. People can
often become confused, require extra nursing attention and, on
occasion, sedation to cope. They may have tests for a variety of
conditions in case these might be contributing to the confusion.
Should they have broken a hip as a consequence of their fall, they
will take longer to rehabilitate because old bones and muscles
take longer to heal. Above all, if they are unlikely to be fit to go
home, it can take many days, weeks, sometimes months to find a
suitable place in residential care or a nursing home.

One hundred years ago these patients would have been looked
after at home, often by family members, recognising that their
predominant need is not for medicine but for care. But social
circumstances have changed remarkably over the last century.
Families are much more geographically dispersed than they used
to be, making it difficult to provide informal support for parents
who are beginning to become frail. Even where children live

closer to their ageing parents, they are often working long hours, with long commuting journeys and do not have much time to provide day-to-day care. Because family size has decreased there are fewer siblings to share the load. They may also fall into the 'sandwich generation' where they not only have ageing parents to worry about, but dependent children as well. Along with these social trends, marriages have become less stable and more families are re-constituted, weakening ties to biological parents.

Older people who are socially isolated and feel lonely are more likely to be admitted to hospital and residential care. Having a tight-knit family may help to prevent this but friends and neighbours are also important. Older people are more likely to maintain their independence and remain healthy if friends or neighbours are popping in to see them on a regular basis and they get the chance to be involved in local activities. Unfortunately, as Robert Putnam's research has shown, many communities have lost these ties of fellowship[25]. It is not ageing on its own that is contributing to the strain on healthcare systems, but also the loss of social ties, which is leading older people to rely more heavily on them.

Young adults too are experiencing an increasing burden of disease. Some of this is as a result of surviving childhood with previously fatal conditions. Cystic fibrosis is a good example, as are some metabolic, blood clotting and immune disorders. A further medical success has been an increase in the survival of very low birth-weight babies. A significant proportion of these children have long-term complications, such as cerebral palsy, requiring a lifetime of care.

Mental health problems often appear for the first time in young adulthood as do the early signs of alcohol and drug dependency. For pregnant women, this can lead to a range of complications, reducing mother and child's life chances as well as creating more demand for healthcare. For other young people it can lead to hospitalisation for acute psychotic illness, injuries sustained whilst under the influence of alcohol or drugs

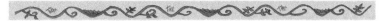

and suicide attempts. Over time these psychological problems can also lead to physical complications like viral hepatitis, skin infections and septicaemia from injecting drug use and liver cirrhosis from long-term excessive alcohol consumption. Many of these conditions require life-long medical monitoring and treatment.

Cultural drivers of ill health in the 21st century

The underlying causes of the shift in the pattern of disease go deep into the culture of modern society. As Zygmunt Baumann has pointed out, we now live "liquid lives" of constant striving and reinvention, with shifting loyalties, identities and beliefs[26]. In the melting pot of late modernity we are having to lead lives in a context riddled with uncertainty and ambiguity, lacking the stability of old. Debates rage between evolutionists and creationists, science and religion, unionists and separatists. Opinion on all things is polarised. Arguments flow around the role of the state and the individual, public and private, targeted or universal benefits, a common good or corporate annexation of territory and resources. In the confusion, when things go wrong, the media assume there must be someone to blame, someone who should have seen this coming, someone who is in charge.

Slow, deep thinking is scarce and attention spans are short. A nagging sense of insecurity and anxiety permeates the airwaves, drowning out wiser, more nuanced voices. In this context maintaining a sense of coherence and a feeling that life is manageable can become difficult, which in turn is having an impact on our health. The changing pattern of 'dis-ease' is a reflection of this confusion and modernist responses are only going to make things worse[27].

To take the obesity epidemic as an example, what we are having to work with is a world of extraordinary complexity in which even apparently simple problems have multiple interlocking causes. As Raj Patel points out in *Stuffed and*

Starved (itself a commentary on the paradox that the obesity epidemic occurs in a world where 12% of people are dangerously undernourished), the world food market is now controlled by a small number of multinational companies who strive hard to protect their market share[28]. These companies spend huge sums marketing and distributing high calorie food and drinks, making them cheap and widely available. Other cultural influences such as the expanding working day and longer commuting journeys reduce the time and inclination to cook meals from scratch. Work is more sedentary. Agricultural practices and subsidies have reduced diversity in modern diets and processing has reduced the quality of micronutrients available. Processed foods are less satisfying and are heavily marketed - "the snack you can eat between meals" - encouraging us to eat more overall. Because of changes in households and people spending considerable amounts of time driving cars, more people eat alone without others to moderate intake. Food becomes a replacement for human intimacy and comfort — the word 'companion' is derived from the Latin *cum panis*, 'with bread', suggesting friendship developing along with sharing meals. The distractions of TV, computers and mobile phones make us less attentive to our eating habits, so we fail to notice our grazing behaviours. In short, our obesity epidemic is not the result of any one factor but a complex interweaving of conditions that together make our culture itself 'obesogenic'[29].

In a similar way, there are many factors which combine to suggest our contemporary culture is also 'addictogenic' — prone to lead us into addictive behaviours. As Bruce Alexander has shown in his book, *The Globalisation of Addiction*, when family and community ties break down, traditional values are undermined and people lose their sense of identity and belonging[30]. People are attracted into addiction as a way of burying their pain, finding a community and a purpose in life, even if the addiction itself is profoundly self-destructive. If these processes are also coupled with widespread de-regulation, opportunities for addiction increase. Relaxed licensing hours for the purchase of alcohol, planning permission for casinos, the easy availability of on-line betting, an explosion of hand-held devices, websites, magazines and channels to cater for every interest, advertising using highly manipulated body images creating dissatisfaction with one's own – all open up the range of possible addictions. Alexander even suggests that in the face of such cultural bombardment from different sources vying for attention, becoming overwhelmingly involved in one activity can be a rational, adaptive response.

The pattern of health inequalities can also be seen as having cultural roots. In their book *The Spirit Level*, Wilkinson and Pickett describe how the widening gap between rich and poor creates more suffering and premature death amongst the poor compared with the more affluent. The scale of this "structural violence" as they describe it contributes to many more deaths than war or pestilence. Wider inequalities in society lead to increasingly socially divisive and segregating policies. This moves public spending away from positive investment in education, infrastructure and sustainable economics to security, correctional facilities and the courts. Between 1984 and 1998 California built twenty-one new prisons but just one new college.

Consumerism and materialism generate further pressures to assert status in an unequal society[31]. People are trapped on a 'hedonic treadmill' working long hours to maintain their living standards with consequent harm to their health and wellbeing.

℮ Reflection

Without stable cultural bearings the world appears less manageable and understandable. Life begins to lose meaning.

This loss of coherence underpins the changing pattern of disease in society today and will not be effectively addressed by existing healthcare systems. I make that claim partly because, as the following chapter shows, the costs are becoming prohibitive. But also because there is a mismatch between the solutions offered by modern medicine, drugs and technologies and the *cultural* scale of the challenges outlined above. Medicine either needs to change to address the new pattern of 'dis-ease' or accept that it is no longer as relevant in dealing with our contemporary health challenges as it used to be. The epidemiological transition from acute to chronic disease has been called the "healthcare equivalent of climate change" — a phrase that carries with it both an idea of the magnitude of the shift and the poverty of our efforts so far to address it[32].

The 'dis-eases' of the 21ˢᵗ century have their origins in the way we live our lives — from pregnancy, through early childhood, to our relationships and culture. The patterning of our lives in terms of our biography is written on our bodies and minds. Treating these 'dis-eases' as if they are bio-mechanical problems of the individual and patching people up when they are in crisis has limited effect. Medical technology cannot provide an effective answer to what are existential problems, related to who we are and how we live rather than to whether our bodies 'work'.

CHAPTER 3

Costing an Arm and a Leg

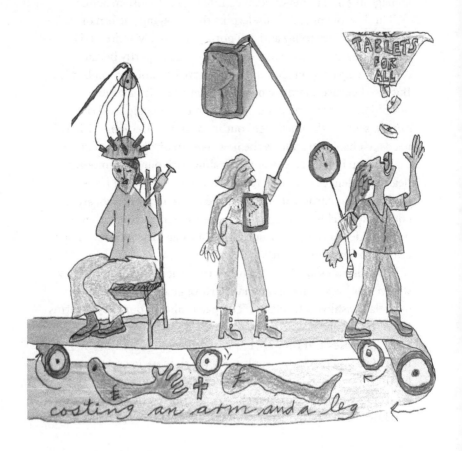

"If something cannot go on forever, it will stop."

Herbert Stein

We turn now to the most obvious symptom of the crisis in healthcare: the seemingly inexorable rise in costs. The trends I have described so far inevitably have consequences in terms of an ever-increasing demand for modern healthcare which also has to be paid for. This is a challenge across the developed world — when in spite of the best efforts of policy makers, think tanks, more or less radical reform programmes and the expensive attention of some of the world's finest management consultants, costs are not only not falling but are increasing at a faster rate than before.

This chapter looks briefly at the main sources of the rise in costs — a phenomenon that now seems embedded in the modern mechanical model itself.

Inexorable demand

Healthcare spending in developed countries around the world has grown exponentially. From 1950 until the financial crash of 2008, the rate of growth in real terms in the UK averaged 4% per year. Before the crash the NHS budget increased in real terms in all but three years of its existence. We seem powerless to stem the tide.

The same pattern of real budget increases, year by year and decade by decade, is replicated across the developed world. Over a thirty year period spending on healthcare across OECD countries has risen from an average of less than $500 per capita to around $3,000 in real terms — a sixfold increase. The dramatic and inexorable rise in spending is astonishing. And the pace of increase has itself been increasing. Within the last twelve years in the UK, for example, spending on healthcare more than doubled from around £50 billion in 1998 to over £120 billion in 2010. This rate of growth is much higher than that of the economy as a whole resulting in healthcare spending comprising 10% of GDP in 2010 compared to just 3% in the 1950s. In the USA it is closer to 17% and rising at roughly 1% per year.

Back in 1948, when the NHS was founded, people never imagined this rise in costs and demand for healthcare. Far from it. They thought that once immediate health concerns were addressed, initial increases in funding for the NHS would level off to steady state: universal access would improve the health of the population and the level of healthcare available would then be sufficient to meet remaining need. Thus, the architect of the NHS, Nye Bevan, reported to Parliament in 1953 that demand for ophthalmic and dental services were in decline, evidence that patient need was being met. However, he was puzzled that despite introducing charges in 1951 the number of prescriptions for drugs had increased. He concluded (presciently) that this must be due to doctors' prescribing behaviour rather than increasing patient demand.

One of the reasons the founders of the NHS thought healthcare costs could be contained was that the post-war government did not just provide universal access to healthcare but also aimed policy and programmes 'upstream' - addressing what Beveridge described in his blueprint for the welfare state as the "Five Giants" of Ignorance, Idleness, Want, Squalor and Sickness. The famous 'post-war consensus' in Britain saw governments of both political persuasions from 1948 to 1979 working to achieve universal access to education, full employment, state pensions, unemployment and sickness benefits and social housing for those who could not afford to buy or rent their own home privately. These were all health-promoting measures at the level of the population.

These policies were highly successful. Better housing reduced the spread of infections such as tuberculosis, which was a big killer before the Second World War. Women's education in particular is linked to the use of contraception and smaller family

size, which has a big impact on population health. Improved
literacy helped people to absorb important health information
– the benefits of booking early with a midwife when pregnant,
getting children vaccinated, etc. Economic policies aimed
to re-distribute the benefits of economic growth. In the UK
corporation tax was introduced in 1965 and the Equal Pay Act in
1970. Income inequalities fell in the post-war era until the late
1970s.

However, since the 1980s, inequalities in the UK have risen
again[33]. Economic growth has continued but so too has growth
in environmental and social costs[34]. As described in the previous
chapter, the post-war consensus has unraveled and the Beveridge
vision has eroded.

Particularly following the financial crash in 2008, many
countries in Europe and elsewhere are cutting back on social
investment, exacerbating inequalities. Higher unemployment,
increasing poverty, debt, overcrowding and pressure to meet
household bills all impact on health, creating more demand
for healthcare and leaving health services struggling to cope.
Now that economic growth has all but ground to a halt in many
developed countries, healthcare spending has become a major
concern.

Medical technology

Macroeconomics is not the only reason for pressure on healthcare
finances today. The rise in prescriptions noted by Bevan has
continued to the present day. At the same time, healthcare
technology has become increasingly sophisticated and the
potential pool of people likely to benefit has grown. The result is
a reinforcing systems loop: demand for increasingly sophisticated
and expensive healthcare is feeding supply and supply is feeding
demand in a process which has come to be known as the 'medical-
industrial complex'[35].

This dynamic is fed by huge advances in medical technology ranging from organ transplantation, joint replacement, reconstructive surgery, anti-cancer drugs to imaging and diagnostics. As these techniques have improved and got safer, more people have become eligible for treatment. And as baby boomers have begun to age there are many more people with age-related degenerative conditions, requiring repair (e.g. coronary arteries) and replacements (e.g. joints and cataracts).

As a result of these modern treatments some previously fatal illnesses can now be cured. A great many more have become chronic. Using figures from Scotland where the number of new cases of heart disease fell by 28% and the death rate by 40% between 2001 and 2010, the result is that the number of people living with heart disease has risen by 70% in the same time period — from roughly 500,000 to 850,000 people[36]. Achieving cure in some cases and extending life in many more is a huge success story for modern medicine but costs go up as more people require on-going treatment for chronic conditions.

The more frequent and widespread use of medical technology also carries the risk of complications which can push up the costs of healthcare. In vitro fertilisation treatment for example often requires more than one fertilised embryo to be put back in the womb. This has the benefit of giving women a greater chance of having a healthy baby, but also increases the chance of twins and triplets. Having twins or triplets carries bigger risks in pregnancy compared with a singleton birth, some of which, such as cerebral palsy, can have lifelong implications[37].

Drugs

A special case of the rise in spending on medical 'technology' is the drugs bill. From the late 1950s to the 1980s there was an explosion in pharmaceutical research with the arrival of many new classes of drug to treat disease. There have been fewer breakthrough therapies since, but a large number of 'me-too'

drugs where companies have made slight modifications and different formulations for existing drugs. In recent years some of the rise in prescribing has been attributable to an ageing population: more people are taking medication, many of them taking several different drugs. Between 2001 and 2011 prescriptions in England rose from 374 to 961 million with the average number of items prescribed per person increasing from just under 12 to over 18 per year[38]. The biggest rises were for anti-depressants, anti-heart disease drugs and treatments for diabetes. Over the same period costs have gone up by over 40% to £8.8 billion — roughly 10% of the overall healthcare budget. The drug industry claims it is controlling costs and indeed prices for many drugs have fallen. Others have come off patent allowing the use of cheaper generic versions. Nevertheless profits remain buoyant through the sheer volume of drugs being prescribed.

Another reason for the rise in prescriptions is closer to Bevan's original supposition: doctors are encouraged to use more of them. This has mostly come about because drugs are being used not just to treat but to prevent disease. The decision to 'treat' is based on protocols drawn up by experts who review the evidence and determine a threshold for prescribing. But drug companies have been keen to fund research to demonstrate the value of their products for prevention and have also worked hard to support the development of guidelines around those they produce. Over time a number of thresholds set in guidelines have been lowered, meaning that more people are prescribed drugs as a preventive measure. This process has become so endemic that being detected with a risk factor such as moderately raised blood pressure or cholesterol has become an illness in itself. People say, "I'm being treated for my cholesterol".

A further reason for this rise in prescriptions is that in the UK doctors are paid for prescribing. Thresholds in their contracts for achieving the necessary levels of 'treatment' vary. They can include ensuring that 80% of patients with high blood pressure

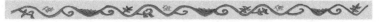

are treated to below a particular blood pressure measurement in order for the practice to earn points to trigger a payment. Ninety percent of patients with a certain risk of heart disease have to be treated with a statin to gain more points and another payment.

There are consequences in the number of drugs being prescribed, not least their potential toxicity. Six percent of hospital admissions in one study have been attributed to adverse drug reactions[39].

A further problem lies with antibiotics as micro-organisms are becoming resistant to their effects. When patients are infected with resistant organisms, they need to be treated with newer, more expensive antibiotics and in many cases kept in isolation until they recover, greatly increasing the costs of treatment and care.

Overdiagnosis

As our healthcare system has become more complex and sophisticated a new phenomenon has become ever more apparent: overdiagnosis. Diagnostic tests carry uncertainty and have the potential to yield positive results which, on further investigation, prove to be false. The chances of a false positive test increase when the background likelihood of real disease is low. This is the situation when you test people who have no symptoms for a disease, such as occurs in population screening programmes. A lot of people who test positive for a screening test have to undergo further investigations to see if it is a true result or not. However, even if further investigation of a positive screening test shows evidence of cancer (usually diagnosed by examining a tissue biopsy), there are difficulties. The body is constantly repairing and regenerating its cells and on occasions this process can become dysfunctional. Cells can appear cancerous when examined under a microscope but later return to normal and not cause any problems. It is impossible to tell from their appearance which ones will spontaneously regress and which ones will progress to harmful cancer so all of these cases are treated the same. The net result is overdiagnosis: people are treated for abnormalities which would not have caused them any harm. Studies suggest that breast cancer screening programmes overdiagnose by 25-50%[40,41].

Overdiagnosis can also occur when people are being tested for other reasons. A scan of the abdomen, pelvis, chest, head or neck can reveal incidental findings in up to 40% of individuals. Some of these are tumours, most of them benign. A very small minority of people might benefit from early detection of an incidental malignant tumour, which was not causing any symptoms. Many others suffer the anxiety and adverse effects of further investigation and treatment of an 'abnormality' that would never have harmed them[42].

As Margaret McCartney points out in her book, *The Patient Paradox*, well people are the health marketeer's dream[43]. Playing on anxieties about cancer, stroke and heart disease, they can be lured into getting tested for "peace of mind". But the effects of overdiagnosis are pernicious. In the words of Iona Heath, former President of the Royal College of General Practitioners:

> "We have, for the first time in history, separated our notions of disease from the human experience of suffering and have created an epidemic of disease without symptoms, defined only by aberrant biometrics. An ever greater proportion of healthcare resources are directed towards reducing these numbers to some fictitious state of normality. In the process, those who are perfectly well are not only assigned labels that in themselves can be shown to compromise health but are also exposed to treatments with significant adverse effects."[44]

Maintaining infrastructure

Roughly 30% of healthcare spending is on infrastructure: the cost of maintaining existing buildings, updating and maintaining staff

skills, investment in IT and repayment of debt. Furthermore, rising fuel costs are putting a strain on budgets through increased heating and transport bills.

In the UK private finance deals have been used to build new hospitals; these have locked the NHS into repayment schemes lasting 30 years or more. Many of these deals were agreed with high rates of interest. The recent squeeze on healthcare spending has meant some hospitals have not been able to cope with the strain of repayments and have needed financial bail-outs.

Staffing

Staff costs contribute roughly 60% of overall healthcare spending. Both staff numbers and staff pay have been increasing. Between 2003 and 2013, the number of consultant doctors rose by 30% in NHS Scotland, GPs by 9% and nurses by 5%. Similar increases have been observed in NHS England, although there was a slight decrease (1%) in overall numbers of staff in 2013 compared wit 2012.

In the early 2000s new contracts were negotiated in the NHS which led to a 15% increase in pay for non-medical staff, a 23% increase for GPs and a 25% increase for hospital consultants. Under these NHS contracts staff were also entitled to annual incremental pay rises, provided they were able to demonstrate that their skills and experience had improved. In an average year this amounts to an additional 2.5% increase in costs for the NHS, an increase which is built into contracts and not something that can be cancelled without lengthy renegotiation.

Independent Pay Review Boards make recommendations for annual pay rises to keep pay in line with inflation. This is a separate process from annual increments. Since 2010 NHS staff have been subject to a pay freeze and have to contribute substantially more to their pensions compared with previous generations of staff. These downward pressures on pay have led to a 12% drop in living standards for healthcare staff over the last three years. This cannot continue indefinitely: inevitably pressure is now growing to allow pay to rise again.

℃ Reflection

While we all want to be treated in the most effective way when we get ill, healthcare has expanded to such an extent that developed nations spend far more on treating illness — whether experienced in the present or possible in the future — than they invest in education, housing, childcare, transport and other infrastructure that enhances the quality of life. If we carry on as we are, healthcare spending will inevitably consume an ever greater proportion of GDP.

The founders of the NHS saw healthcare as part of a wider welfare programme which aimed to reduce poverty and poor housing, raise education standards and achieve full employment. Protecting healthcare spending at the expense of these other dimensions of social welfare during economic austerity could well exacerbate ill health – the very problem healthcare aims to address.

From a macroeconomic systems perspective, maintaining high levels of spending on healthcare when other government spending is cut to the bone is a fix that will fail. We desperately need to take a wider view of the problem if we are to escape this simplistic focus on budgets — a problem that decades of failure suggest we cannot solve.

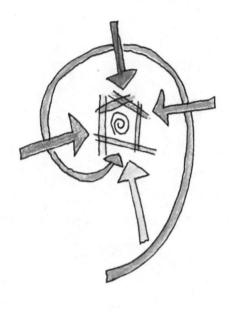

PART 2:
THE RESPONSE

Chapter 4

The Brakes are Failing

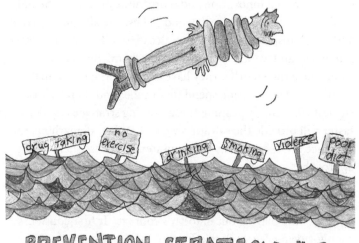

drug taking   no exercise   drinking   smoking   violence   poor diet

PREVENTION STRATEGY #5

"All systems face challenges — and none of them have fully figured out the formula for providing high-quality universal care at a cost that is sustainable over the long haul."
Peter Behner, *Strategy and Business*, August 2011

The recent financial crisis has placed an enforced constraint on healthcare budgets which had previously continued to rise in spite of our best efforts to contain them. In the UK we are now facing flat-line budgets for the foreseeable future, even as demand for healthcare — as we have seen — continues to rise.

The response has been to redouble efforts to increase efficiency, find cost savings, increase productivity, look for savings through innovation and reorganisation and — the holy grail — attempt to reduce demand. These are all familiar, tried and tested responses from recent decades. Of course they are important and we should not abandon them. But likewise we should face the fact that they have been insufficient to make any significant dent in rising spend for decades and there is little to suggest that simply pushing these existing strategies harder and faster will provide the salvation we seek today. If anything, the evidence is the opposite — the unintended consequences of these approaches actually make the system more fragile, less resilient and draw it inexorably closer to collapse.

This chapter explores in more detail how these existing strategies are playing out in today's context. It first considers supply-side measures then efforts to influence demand.

Supply-side strategies

With costs rising, healthcare systems have explored and prosecuted a number of strategies to get them back under control. On the supply-side these have largely been inspired by tried and tested strategies from business and industry — 'lean' efficiency savings, streamlining 'back-office' functions, investing in 'labour-saving' IT, encouraging competition to drive

down costs. Each strategy is familiar and continues to have its advocates (more so now than ever). But in the complex setting of contemporary healthcare these simple interventions are not only losing efficiency they are now showing significant negative side-effects. A sample of the most popular strategies follows.

Staff costs

Healthcare provision is labour intensive with staff costs accounting for some 60% of healthcare budgets. Inevitably the search for savings alights first on staff costs. Vacancies are left open, staff not replaced when they retire, the level of training needed to perform a role is reduced. In the UK, healthcare workers have been subject to a pay freeze for several years and are being required to pay more into their pension schemes. Back-office functions have been centralised and combined wherever possible creating further opportunities to reduce staffing levels. Elsewhere in Europe (for example, Greece, Ireland, Spain) where the Eurozone crisis has been particularly severe, staff are not being paid for months on end or are being laid off altogether.

Sooner or later these strategies have an impact on the quality of care. Doing more for less leaves those still in jobs taking on wider responsibilities with less support from managers or senior clinicians. Staff are leaving — retiring early, emigrating to other countries or becoming ill under the strain. New people coming into post quickly lose confidence, thinking they are incompetent in not managing their workload, whereas in reality the job they have been recruited to do is itself unmanageable. Part of the reason for this is that staff cuts fall disproportionately on managers and administrative staff in an effort to protect 'the frontline'. This often ends up being a false economy as clinical staff find themselves doing managerial tasks for which they have little or no training whilst reducing their face-to-face time with people who are ill and in need of their expertise.

Information Technology

Also near the top of the list for cost savings and 'rationalisation' is the introduction of new technology to automate systems, share data and generally increase efficiency. This approach has a poor track record in healthcare, where attempts at developing national systems, so that everyone is sharing one electronic record for example, have ended up costing far more money than expected. Where these projects are finally implemented, local providers of healthcare can find themselves locked into unwieldy mainframe solutions. Often it requires a skilled administrator to manage and interrogate these systems and make the necessary connections to other systems so that laboratory investigations, appointments, reminders, etc. can all be linked to one patient. People are constantly moving in and out of geographical areas, requiring information to move from one local system to another. The dream of connecting all this up into a single system for the English NHS (a programme called Connecting for Health) was eventually abandoned, but not until more than £10 billion had been spent.

Increased competition

As funding constraints have grown more intense there has been a drive towards opening up more of the health service to market forces, particularly in the English NHS. If drug companies and other suppliers to the health service are governed by market forces and have been the biggest innovators in health care, then why not introduce more competition into the health service itself? Surely this will trigger more cost savings and efficiency gains?

For high volume, single treatment procedures such as cataract surgery or hip replacements, private providers may well be able to undercut the NHS on price. However, the funding for healthcare in the UK comes from general taxation and is allocated to local areas on a per capita basis. If a private provider is selected to supply cataract surgery to a population the money that goes to the provider is taken from the existing service. The original service still has to provide eye surgery for other purposes — correcting squints, treating traumatic injuries, etc. but has far less money to pay for its staff. This may lead to one or two surgeons not being replaced when they leave or retire, and providing the service 365 days a year becomes impossible. If there is no eye surgeon, providing a comprehensive trauma service becomes problematic. This in turn might lead to other services becoming undermined and people having to travel further for treatment. Local hospital provision breaks up.

The point here is that health services are a tightly coupled web of interacting providers. Redirecting one small stream of activity into an alternative provider may make sense for a short-term efficiency gain, but can be highly disruptive of the system as a whole.

Consolidation of services

Another option, as the drive for efficiency savings continues, is consolidating services in fewer sites. Rather than leave this to the vagaries of the market, might there be other ways to take into account the wider system and rationalise services in a co-ordinated way? After all, there are good clinical reasons for creating centres of excellence where surgeons and doctors are familiar with complex procedures and can carry them out safely and reliably.

In practice these consolidations are extremely difficult given that they have to accommodate multiple stakeholder interests. They often take years to implement, requiring extensive public involvement if the clinical case is to be understood. The situation has worsened in England where new legislation means mergers have to be referred to the Competition Commission to review their effect on a competitive market for healthcare[45]. Meanwhile, cost pressures build and hospital finances are stretched to breaking point.

In market-based health economies providers can go to the wall because there will be others to take their place. Competition implies some duplication of services which builds in a level of redundancy that allows (indeed expects) individual providers to fail. This brings with it a financial premium and goes some way to explaining the high cost of healthcare in the US, where cities in particular are heavily over-supplied with hospitals.

As a centrally-planned health economy, the NHS has no such redundancy in hospital provision. When a provider gets into a dire financial state its hospitals cannot close because they are still needed to provide essential healthcare to the population. In 2012 South London NHS Trust was put under special administration because it was losing £1 million a day largely because of debt repayments. Despite huge efforts to generate savings, it was not turning this around. In 2013 the organisation was dissolved, its hospitals taken over by other local providers and its debts paid by the government. The cost of this bail-out for the taxpayer was £466 million[46].

Limiting demand

If we cannot control costs, clearly we need to limit demand. This is the attraction of market-based models of health care, in which the price mechanism can both regulate demand and provide

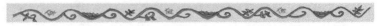

incentives in the system to reduce it (stay healthy to avoid the cost, or to gain insurance discounts for example). In a 'universal' system, such as the UK, the proxy for this approach is rationing. Like the methods for cost control, these strategies flow for the most part from seeing healthcare as a product or a service industry like any other. Slightly more sophisticated is the public health agenda of prevention and health promotion — which at least has a foothold in health-related knowledge and expertise even if it too now appears more like a branch of modeling or behavioural economics. These strategies — and their drawbacks — are described briefly below.

Rationing through eligibility criteria and charges

The most obvious way to reduce demand in a service that provides 'universal' access is to look at the eligibility criteria for particular treatments. In some parts of the UK, funders now stipulate the limits of movement and pain needed to get a hip or knee replacement. These measures fail to take into account individual circumstances. A hip replacement might be needed at a lower level of pain and limitation of movement if a person has an active job, requiring them to be on their feet all day, compared with someone who has retired and is able to do most things that they want. An even more bizarre situation has arisen in some areas where the minimum Body Mass Index required to be eligible for the gastric band operation has increased. There is now an incentive for patients to put on weight to get their operation for weight loss!

As the financial crisis deepens, the call for introducing more charges for the use of healthcare grows. There are several problems with this idea: it penalises people when they are sick; it is regressive as poor people are more likely to be sick and flat rate payments hit them hard; the cost of administering such schemes is high; and it flies in the

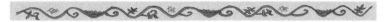

face of the original aim of the NHS which was to provide healthcare through funding from central taxation.

There is a counter-argument which suggests that free healthcare can have perverse incentives. For example, free prescriptions which are available to people in Scotland and Wales and to many who are exempt from charges in England reduce options for promoting healthy lifestyles as a way of combating ill health. It might be more beneficial for someone to exercise regularly at a leisure centre to control their blood pressure than take a pill. But the medication is free for the patient while the entrance fee to the centre is not. Some areas have devised schemes whereby doctors can provide an 'exercise prescription' but they are paid for through separate funding rather than by diverting some of the prescribing budget.

Prevention strategies

Public health has a long history of taking action to improve health and prevent disease. Pioneers of public health worked to provide clean water and sanitation in the 19th century and eliminated the regular cholera outbreaks in industrialising cities around the world. In the first half of the 20th century public health campaigners achieved better health for women and children through contraception, access to maternity services and child vaccination programmes. They continue to advocate good housing, universal access to health care and education, redistribution of wealth and greater public involvement in decision-making to create the enabling conditions for better health.

Many chronic diseases today are linked to behaviours — smoking, drinking, poor diet, lack of exercise, drug-taking and violence. Public health has had some success with reducing smoking – campaigning to ban advertising of tobacco products and increasing the age at which they can be purchased, creating smoke-free public places and providing support for people wanting to quit. Smoking in Britain fell from about 80% in men and 40% in women in 1950 to 20% in both sexes in 2010. This has been matched by a marked reduction in lung cancer among men and it is beginning to decline among women.

Given this success, maybe the same measures for controlling promotion, and access, and providing support for those who want to change their behaviour could reduce drinking and drug taking, improve eating habits, increase physical activity and reduce violence? There are many calls to do this: regulate the current market mechanisms for alcohol (minimum pricing, licensing), fizzy drinks (a soda tax) and fast food (ban advertising to children) and provide support for people who escape from violent relationships. All these can improve health and reduce illness. There is evidence that they may have some impact on consumption. De-criminalisation and improving access to addiction services would help reduce harm from illicit drug-taking which remains highly hazardous as an outbreak of anthrax in injecting drug users in Scotland in 2009 and 2010 demonstrated. There were 119 cases and 14 deaths. Health Protection Scotland, which led the investigation, warned in its report on the outbreak that as long as there is an illegal drug trade, this danger would remain.

Physical activity can be encouraged through designing and building environments which encourage children to play and people to walk and cycle rather than use the car. They have other benefits in terms of social interaction, clean air and reduced carbon emissions. The social environment can also be shaped with the provision of quality family centres, parental leave and allowances.

All these strategies offer some benefits in reducing the demand for health services but many of them fail to address the inter-connectedness of these complex problems. In real life, it is not uncommon to find people smoking, drinking, taking drugs, eating badly, taking no exercise, providing chaotic parenting and living in violent relationships. These people are heavy users of health services, often through Accident and Emergency and into hospital care. There are other consequences for their children who often get taken into care, underperform at school and not infrequently end up in the criminal justice system. There are no easy answers.

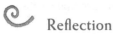 Reflection

The current orthodoxy about efficiency savings and competition seems to be the only game in town: it effectively closes down any serious debate about more radical options for moving to sustainable, effective healthcare. The debate assumes we can marshal our limited resources in smarter and smarter ways in order to meet rising demand. That looks like a slim hope. Stripping out inefficiencies may work for one or two years, but not for ten.

Current efficiency measures fail to take into account the complexity of what we are dealing with. Holding posts vacant and applying a pay freeze keeps the books balanced (or at least holds the debt at a viable level) but wears staff down over time. Sickness absence and early retirement levels rise, leaving critical decisions to be made by inexperienced staff. Preventive strategies are fragmented and unlikely to have a systemic impact on demand for healthcare any time soon.

So how can we expect to maintain quality in a system under this much pressure? It is to that issue that we must now turn.

CHAPTER 5

Regulation, Inspection and the Fight Against Error

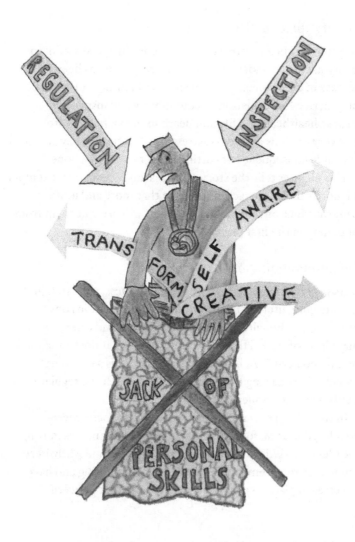

> *"Even if good care strives after good results, the quality of care*
> *cannot be deduced from its results. Instead, what characterises*
> *good care is a calm, persistent but forgiving effort to improve*
> *the situation of a patient, or to keep this from deteriorating."*
>
> Anne Marie Mol, *The Logic of Care*, 2008

Quality under pressure

As systems of healthcare have come under financial strain, so
quality has come under pressure. The response has been an
increase in the frequency, detail and assiduousness of structures
and practices of regulation, accountability and inspection.
Because healthcare is a life and death industry, failures are
both very obvious and very distressing. Yet in part they are an
inevitable consequence of cutting the service to the bone.

This chapter tells the story of increasingly desperate attempts
to ignore this simple fact in the hope that more and more
stringent sanctions for making mistakes will prevent them from
happening in the first place.

Regulating professionals

By its very nature, healthcare is a risky business, with staff and
patients quite literally facing life and death situations on a
routine basis. Equally, treatments carry risks and often require
a high level of skill. Hippocrates cautioned that doctors should
"first do no harm". Achieving this in practice is a constant
struggle. Formalising the principle started with the regulation of
healthcare practitioners.

In the UK, national standards required of doctors were
introduced in 1858, for midwives in 1902 and for nurses in 1919.
The General Medical Council and the Nursing and Midwifery
Council set requirements for education and training and have
processes in place to deal with fitness to practice concerns.

Regulation tended to place the primary responsibility for safety with professionals themselves.

This reliance on professional self-regulation was brought into sharp focus with the case of Harold Shipman in the UK. A general practitioner for twenty-four years, Shipman was found guilty in 2000 of killing fifteen patients. The police investigation suggested he probably killed around 250 people making him one of the most prolific serial killers in recorded history. The case shocked the nation and led to a thorough review of death certification. Regulation of doctors was tightened up. Through a process of revalidation they are now re-certified as fit to practice every five years. Nursing too has had its scandals. Beverly Allitt, a nurse on a children's ward, was found guilty of murdering four children, attempting to murder three more and causing grievous bodily harm on a further six in 1993. These are dramatic cases in which individuals abuse their power when people are at their most vulnerable.

Every system will have some people operating with malicious intent who will need to be brought to book. Far more common are accidents, mistakes and healthcare associated infections which can lead to deaths and complications, generate complaints and sometimes lead to claims for negligence. Litigation costs have risen by 40% in five years to more than £1.2 billion in England in 2012.

The risks of healthcare

If Florence Nightingale were to return to a hospital today, what would she make of it? She would be astonished by the cars filling the car park, ambulances turning up at Accident and Emergency and countless different types of electronic device being used — phones, monitors, diagnostic instruments. However, once she made it up on to a ward, there would still be many things she would recognise — a nurses' station, beds in bays, monitoring charts for temperature, blood pressure and pulse. The underlying culture of healthcare is much as it was 100 years ago — the clinical assessment of a problem by a trained doctor, a treatment regime prescribed and nursing care provided where needed.

Nightingale might also start to notice the strain on the system. Because of the cost pressures described in previous chapters and the subsequent efficiency savings that have been extracted by reducing hospital beds and staffing numbers, services run close to maximum capacity most of the time. Patients are discharged much more quickly than they used to be, the ward is often noisy, nurses have less time to get to know patients and spend a lot of time on paperwork recording what is happening to them as they come and go. Junior doctors work in rotations, handing over complex cases at regular intervals and rarely see a patient through the course of their illness. As the pace and volume of work through hospitals and other health settings grows, so too does the risk of something going wrong.

Equipment supplies can also create problems. Contamination of blood products created an outbreak of HIV in France. Injectable steroid led to an outbreak of meningitis in the USA. Breast implants contaminated with poor quality silicone have ruptured. When these incidents occur, huge efforts are needed to investigate the cause, stop further harm and learn lessons for the future. When public scrutiny is intense this can be fraught and stressful for everyone involved even before the courts get involved.

Maintaining the safety of healthcare systems is in itself a time-consuming and costly business. Drugs have to be given within their expiry date, equipment sterilised, hands washed whenever staff are in direct contact with patients as well as at other points of care. Intravenous lines need setting up, wounds need to be kept clean and dressed, bed-bound patients turned regularly — which all requires vigilance. Under pressure in a high-paced environment, mistakes happen.

As a result, patient safety has become a science and discipline in its own right. Using techniques developed in the airline and other high-risk industries, healthcare has instigated a number of reliable routines to reduce the chances of error. Safety protocols are very effective in highly repetitive, high-risk situations. A pre-operative checklist has been shown to save lives. This ensures that basic information about the person about to have surgery is correct (name, operation, side of body or limb to be operated on, etc.). Just as important, the checklist routine encourages everyone in the team to have a voice, creating a stronger safety culture.

In addition to patient safety initiatives, healthcare organisations have extensive risk management systems. They identify risks, assign a score, develop an action plan to manage the risk and publish a risk register updated on a regular basis. If an incident does occur – a patient falls out of bed, the wrong dose of drug is given, the same surgical instruments are used in consecutive procedures – a review is undertaken and a report written. To maintain transparency and accountability, this work is reported regularly to clinical governance committees and where necessary to complaints offices and solicitors.

What would Florence Nightingale make of the growth in the safety and risk management procedures? In her time the ward sister would have been responsible for the cleanliness and safe running of her ward with the spectre of censure from the hospital matron if this were inadequate. Personal commitment and dedication to the highest standards of care would have made the sister ensure that all was in good order on the ward. The emphasis was on professional accountability.

Now healthcare is a system operating at high pace and under extreme pressure. Put into a highly stressed and understaffed environment, human beings will begin to falter. Checklists and protocols may mitigate the worst aspects of this strain, but where staffing levels are cut to the bone and supervision is scarce, people will cut corners, leading to neglect and compromising standards.

The rise in investigations of professional performance is not the result of a few bad apples but of many bad barrels creaking under the strain.

Regulation — and its consequences

In an attempt to address these concerns, healthcare as a whole – not just individual professionals – has become increasingly regulated. In 1999 the Care Commission was established in England with the aim of advising hospitals and community health services on setting up clinical governance structures. These were designed to monitor practice to ensure patient safety standards were maintained and services learned from their mistakes. Over the following ten years the Care Commission evolved to become the Care Quality Commission. The CQC is no longer merely advisory, but scrutinises many different aspects of healthcare activity. It has powers to call healthcare providers to account should they fall significantly below agreed standards. Inspection reports are published and, if negative, can receive widespread publicity.

Florence Nightingale was a pioneer in collating and analysing hospital statistics, but I suspect she would be surprised at how much scrutiny of healthcare takes place today. No matter how thorough the preparations for inspection (which can involve considerable time away from providing direct care to patients) anxiety levels run high until the visiting team has submitted its report and the service is said to meet the necessary standards. Increasingly these inspections are unannounced, which leaves staff in a constant state of high alert. This may be good in the short term to ensure safety protocols are followed and standards of cleanliness are maintained. However, with finances stretched many hospitals are running wards constantly one or two staff short. Rather than understand the systemic drivers and the threat they pose for clinical standards, inspections put a great strain on staff, inducing a culture of fear and blame.

A pattern is emerging where layers of regulation have been added into the healthcare system in an effort to restore and maintain the quality of care but each layer of regulation is both adding to strain in the system and itself showing signs of strain. Individual complaints by patients and their relatives are rising, leading in turn to more compensation pay-outs. Concerns by employers and the police over fitness for practice have grown exponentially leading to more investigations and hearings for doctors and nurses. Regulatory bodies are struggling to cope with the demands being made of them.

Ensuring timely access to healthcare

In addition to issues of safety and quality are concerns about access to healthcare and, in the UK, the politically sensitive issue of waiting lists (the number of people waiting for an operation) and waiting times (the length of time people have to wait to get seen and treated).

Waiting times cover different points along the pathway of care such as time spent waiting for an ambulance to come following an emergency call, time waiting to be seen in Accident and Emergency and the overall time from referral for a problem by a general practitioner to getting it treated. The stakes are high for hospitals and managers to maintain their required targets and pressure can grow to 'game' the system so that figures for performance on these measures disguise the reality on the ground.

Once a threshold is crossed where it is OK to manipulate the figures, a culture can set in which loses touch with reality and denies the existence of genuine concerns. Such are the lessons from the inquiry into standards of care at Mid-Staffordshire Hospital Trust. In 2005 Mid-Staffordshire was striving to become a Foundation Trust. To do this the hospital had to achieve certain financial as well as performance targets. This resulted in them leaving vacant a large number of posts to save money whilst moving patients from Accident and Emergency into holding areas where they received no clinical care, simply to enable them to achieve the four-hour waiting time target for A&E. Hospital management ignored concerns about standards of care, which judging from the accounts of patients and relatives were deeply shocking. Some patients were so thirsty they were forced to drink water from flower vases, people were left naked and in their own excrement for many hours and bells were left unanswered. Whilst there were many doctors and nurses who continued to provide good quality care at the hospital, many were also subsequently the subject of investigation. Five nurses have been struck off the Nursing and Midwifery Register. Many more have been suspended or cautioned.

In response to concerns at Mid-Staffordshire Hospital the UK government commissioned Don Berwick, founder of the Institute of Healthcare Improvement, to review recommendations in the Francis Report which was produced following an inquiry. Berwick's report, published in 2013, calls for a shift in culture in the NHS from blame to learning. However, unless this culture shift is accompanied by deeper questioning of assumptions about the purpose and intent of modern healthcare, the challenges to the quality of care inherent in a system operating beyond its limits will remain.

Integrity under strain

Meeting targets, making efficiency savings and surviving the latest inspection all sap energy, occupy attention and fail to achieve the results staff are yearning for. Hospital staff are being pressured by the system in which they work to manipulate appointment times to save money and to maintain the illusion that waiting times are being achieved. Some staff are resigning in disgust. Others can't wait to leave. Meanwhile the underlying purpose and integrity of the health service is disintegrating, which will carry a high price in the longer term.

The crisis is no less in other settings beyond the hospital, for example in primary care. Here general practitioners are frustrated by the demands placed on them — both to fulfil various quotas to achieve the necessary targets which will guarantee their income and by the patients themselves, whose attendances grow each year. Ten-minute appointments are inadequate to address the complexity of people's illness, yet inevitable to cope with the workload. The relentless pressure is pushing increasing numbers of doctors to reduce their hours or take early retirement.

Working in this environment is alienating. How can staff who themselves feel drained and exhausted restore patients to health? What is a priority for the manager when everything feels like a priority? Can a GP stop prescribing a drug of marginal benefit to a person if the practice as a result then loses money it needs to employ a nurse?

A health service where everyone is watching their backs, where targets distract from patient care and staff fear losing their jobs if they speak up, provides no space for the creativity and innovation so desperately needed. The disconnection between the aspirations of staff to provide great care and the demands of the system for efficiency generates dissonance, which no amount of restructuring will address. In this climate it can be difficult for staff to retain their sense of purpose and their integrity.

Most people working in health services are drawn to the sector because they care and want to help other people when they are suffering. But the environment of modern healthcare puts such an intolerable burden of demands on them that they find it almost impossible to keep going. In an industrialised system of care staff can feel like very small cogs in a huge machine and work can become mechanical and exhausting. The deep calling to work with people who are sick, injured or frail is undermined.

Clare Gerada (former Chair of the Royal College of General Practitioners in the UK) has described the NHS as experiencing "institutionalised anxiety". This atmosphere is counter-productive: patients are very sensitive to the mood of the

clinicians caring for them and will not be reassured by people under obvious stress themselves. Fearful organisations are not positive therapeutic environments. Patient safety programmes and making good use of practical cues to ensure repetitive tasks are completed reliably ameliorates the worst dangers of this compromised culture, but unless these deeper fears are addressed, the system will continue to degrade.

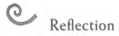

Reflection

The real crisis in healthcare is not financial, but human. Squeezing efficiency out of people generates distress and resentment whilst laying the blame on individuals is not helpful. Recognising the healthcare challenge as fundamentally a human one opens up new avenues for exploration because human systems are special: they are self-aware, creative, intentional and have the potential to transform. But we are unlikely to be able to access that capacity if we continue to treat healthcare as a product and staff as an overhead, not to be trusted.

CHAPTER 6

RCTs: A Self-Limiting Improvement Methodology

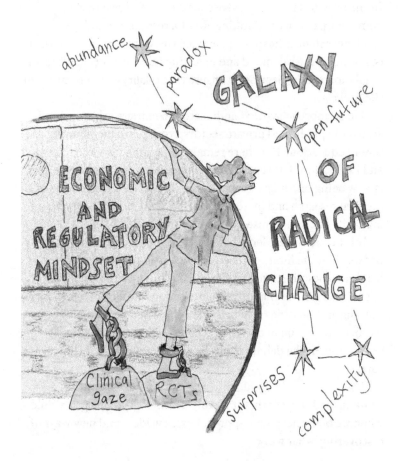

> *"It is axiomatic that the theoretic framework within which we*
> *formulate our research questions determines the scope, content*
> *and social relevance of our answers."*
> Anthony McMichael, 1999[47]

Painting ourselves into a corner

In the previous two chapters we have reviewed two of the
dominant patterns of thinking about a response to today's
challenges in healthcare — managing the system better to reduce
costs and temper demand and investing in robust mechanisms of
regulation and inspection to ensure that quality does not suffer in
the process.

These approaches are familiar from countless other examples
across the public and private sectors, from car manufacturing to
school education. But there remains one further source of reward
and innovation that is particular to medicine and healthcare, and
is now being taken up in other areas. This is the cornerstone of
medical research and increasingly of all 'evidence-based policy
making': the Randomised Controlled Trial (RCT).

It is becoming evident that the RCT methodology itself
has reached the limits of its effectiveness in the contemporary
landscape described in Part One of this book. Even so, it still
has an iron grip on the infrastructure of medical research and its
funding and — aside from orthodox neo-liberal economics —
has become the main currency accepted, carrying authority or
conviction, in the debate about healthcare reform and clinical
care.

This chapter will highlight the blindspots in this way of
thinking and suggest that it is dangerously self-limiting at a time
when we badly need new approaches, new ideas and new ways of
discovering 'what works'.

Does medicine work?

The biggest question we want to know about medicine is whether or not a treatment will work. Traditionally doctors and their patients have judged this on the basis of personal experience — did they get better or not? Gradually, through careful observation, evidence from individual cases of treatment has accumulated and become more systematised. In the early days of medicine much of this work grew through custom and practice and was not subject to objective scientific methods.

This changed radically from the middle of the 20th century with the development of (RCTs) which were designed to prove statistically the benefits of treatments and detect those which caused harm and should therefore be stopped.

A controlled trial studies the effect of a treatment in one group of patients compared with another group of patients (the control) who do not receive it. There are various ways in which a difference might be found between the two groups simply because of the way patients were selected for the treatment and non-treatment groups. Randomisation counteracts this effect. When the two groups are of sufficient size to rule out a difference between them simply by chance, the size of an observed effect of a treatment compared to non-treatment can be considered attributable to the treatment and not to other factors.

The first RCT was undertaken in 1948 to assess the value of the new drug streptomycin in treating tuberculosis. Prior to drug treatment, TB carried a high death rate. In this study just over 100 patients were recruited and allocated randomly to receive streptomycin or a dummy treatment. After six months more than one in four of those not treated had died compared with less than one in ten of those on treatment. It was an impressive clinical result for a novel treatment demonstrating a big effect (significant reduction in the proportion of deaths) in a short space of time (six months).

Evidence accumulated in this way has re-shaped medicine over the last fifty years. As far as possible when new technologies or treatments appear they are tested usually against a placebo (dummy treatment) or less frequently, the existing treatment. If, using statistical methods to analyse the results, a clinically important effect is demonstrated, the new treatments are put to use. Similarly, in some cases existing treatments have been tested using RCTs and stopped when results demonstrate they do not work.

The side effects of Randomised Controlled Trials

But there are problems with this approach. To begin with, recruitment into RCTs is a fraught business. Usually trials are set up to assess the effectiveness of a relatively simple intervention for a particular disease such as coronary artery disease or asthma. But arriving at a diagnosis can be problematic with the result that many people with illness (the kind who often go to see their GPs) will be excluded because their symptoms do not match exactly the diagnostic entry requirements. By restricting entry criteria to those with clear-cut symptoms of a specific disease, clinical research builds up evidence around people who are not representative of the population in the GP's surgery.

Many people are excluded from trials because they also have other conditions, not just the one disease that the researchers are interested in. With so-called 'multi-morbidity' an increasing feature of clinical practice, this is a big exclusion. There may be others. In many early trials for heart disease only middle-aged men were included. Because of the ethical issues surrounding research on children, far fewer RCTs have been conducted in paediatrics than in adult specialties.

Furthermore, many modern drugs do not have the dramatic effect of anti-TB drugs. As a consequence very large numbers of people have to be recruited to demonstrate statistically significant effects. If the research is looking to assess whether

the treatment can reduce long-term complications from chronic disease, trials can require many years of follow-up. This is a costly process and often fraught with uncertainty. Because of these difficulties researchers look for differences in surrogate end-points — a change in blood pressure or sugar levels in the blood rather than a reduction in clinically relevant complications such as heart attacks or amputations.

Clearly, the longer a trial lasts the more difficult it becomes to keep track of everyone involved. Despite the intensive work involved in follow-up, people drop out. This trend has increased over the last 10 years as people have become more aware of their rights to discontinue in research trials and are less trustful of healthcare providers. But missing data can also hide 'a multitude of sins' leaving a doubt over how effective the treatment will be in routine practice[48].

Even with clear-cut results, translating research into practice can be tricky. To begin with, research conclusions need to be made at an agreed cut-off point. In the TB example mentioned above this was six months and the results of treatment with streptomycin were impressive. However, over the course of the next six months many of the treated group got worse again and some died because the infection had grown resistant to streptomycin. It took many more years of trial and error to find a combination of drugs which achieved recovery from the infection whilst avoiding relapse because of drug resistance.

In addition, the clinical team developing this programme had to find the best way to keep an eye on people to make sure they took the drugs for the necessary time period and did not experience serious side effects. In other words, the research phase often needs to be expanded by many more years of embedding the findings in practice before the benefits of a drug or treatment can be fully realised. Yet research funders are configured to support novel research bids with far less attention and funding available for the absorption of new findings into routine care.

Interpreting the numbers

Because of its reliance on statistics, clinical research is largely based on quantitative studies, which rely on the power of big numbers to demonstrate the effect of treatment. But something important is lost — the unique identity of any one patient, or the particular healthcare encounter in which a treatment is initiated.

In other words, quantification which takes place in clinical trials intensifies the 'clinical gaze' described in Chapter 1. Only treatments which are done to people can be assessed. The patient is passive in the extreme. By their design, resources that individuals bring to their own recovery and the unique relationship each one will have with their doctors are excluded.

Because they are reliant on statistical analysis to prove their worth, the particular benefits of a treatment for a particular patient are based on probabilities. Put simply, if a patient asks "Will the treatment work doctor?" the honest reply is "I don't know. All I can say is that studies suggest if a number of people with your condition and no other take this medicine, one of them will get better because of it and not because they would have got better anyway." The actual number of people needing to take a drug for a given benefit will vary depending on what that drug is and the underlying condition it is aiming to treat.

The value of RCTs is that they have been able to quantify the benefit of drugs given to treat illness and prevent complications and disease. It is good to know that if I take a drug, there is a one in five chance it will save my life. It may be comforting to know that I have a one in 122 chance of preventing a heart attack or stroke if I take a drug for my blood pressure for five years even if it does not reduce my overall risk of dying. The downside to this approach, which forms the foundation of evidence-based medicine, is that many people are taking medicines which will not benefit them and may even cause them harm.

Being evidence-based gives medicine *consistency* in practice, but not necessarily *efficacy*. In reality, clinical research can only offer an approximation to the likely effect of a treatment in routine practice. Evidence-based medicine offers a starting point for treatment, but medical practice requires careful attention to people's individual responses and the relationship within which this takes place.

Summarising the results

As clinical research expands, more and more trials are yielding results. Doctors have studied every organ and system in the body, created diagnostic devices of technological brilliance and generated results from hundreds of thousands of research studies accumulating evidence of effectiveness in highly controlled conditions. No doctor can know everything of relevance from this research. The pace of research papers being published far outstrips the human capacity to read and understand them.

In an effort to bring some overall sense to this picture, researchers have developed methods to collate and combine findings from multiple studies which have looked at the same area of treatment in an attempt to summarise the evidence. These methods are called 'systematic reviews' and 'meta-analyses' and have become a research industry in their own right. The National Institute for Health and Care Excellence in England (NICE) is commissioned to review evidence from the literature and consult with stakeholders and the wider public to derive protocols for doctors to follow in the identification and treatment of many different conditions. In the USA insurance companies do something similar when they set out the treatments that can be funded on their policies.

But even what is published as clinical research is open to major doubt. As Ben Goldacre has pointed out, drug companies, who fund a great deal of this research, stand to lose income if a new drug is not as powerful or effective as they had hoped[49]. As a result companies actively suppress studies which show negative or equivocal results for their products so only the more promising ones get published. In addition, researchers are less motivated to write up studies which yield negative results adding further to 'publication bias'. As a result, systematic reviews are subject to the same bias and unless researchers go to extra lengths to seek out these unpublished studies, their results are far from definitive.

Des Spence, writing in the *British Medical Journal* in 2014 asks, "How many people care that the research pond is polluted, with fraud, sham diagnosis, short term data, poor regulation, surrogate ends, questionnaires that can't be validated, and statistically significant but clinically irrelevant outcomes?". It is deeply undermining of medical confidence that the research base on which it relies has become so contaminated.

The clinical research industry is like a juggernaut set on its course because it knows no other. But with vast sums of research money and commercial revenues in play, big research institutions, professorial chairs, public honours and awards all tied into this research infrastructure there is no incentive to call it into question.

The pattern of disease is changing, making the biomechanical model less fit for the task of diagnosis or treatment. Joints wear out through excess weight gain, poor nutrition and low levels of exercise, for example. Whilst clinical research can improve the quality of the device implanted or determine the best surgical technique to use, it has yet to find ways to deal with the increasing demand for joint replacements. Clinical research in its current form squeezes out the possibility of investing in different perspectives, other forms of research or other paradigms for investigation and innovation to tackle our deeply rooted health problems.

ℰ Reflection

So far, I have argued that the clinical, economic and regulatory
mindset which has dominated the healthcare debate is running
out of ideas to deal with the challenges we face. The orthodoxy
has a model of reality, has derived data from this model and has
used these data to drive decisions. It fixes its gaze on what it sees
as quantifiable and objective and excludes other perspectives.
Its reliance on clinical research evidence despite its limitations
makes it hostage to a world based on probabilities rather than the
messy reality of an open future. What's missing is a recognition of
the abundance and complexity of real life, which offers surprises,
paradox and the potential for more radical change.

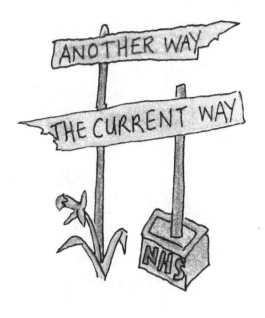

PART 3:

ANOTHER WAY IS POSSIBLE

CHAPTER 7

The Patterning of Hope

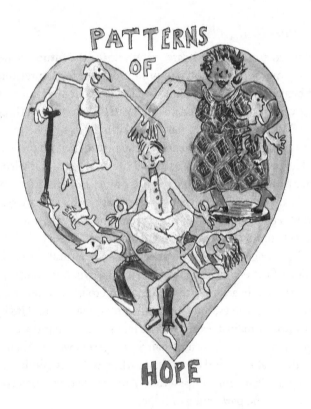

*"The NHS is like an established church, with rigid doctrines, a
well rehearsed liturgy, an army of priests and altar boys and
cathedrals in the form of hospitals, paid for under Private
Finance Initiatives. It begs for a Martin Luther to nail his 95
theses to the door. It hasn't found one yet."*

Nigel Hawkes, *British Medical Journal*, 24 April 2010

The future is already here

If we are to create a healthcare system fit for the future we need
to widen our field of vision to embrace our deeper aspirations for
what healthcare could become. To a large extent staff know that
the current system is unsustainable. Patients want something
better. When asked (and I have asked hundreds of staff and
patients) many have grave fears for the future if we go on as we
are. The pressures and strains are all too apparent. But with
further probing, it is possible to hear a more hopeful story and
to find existing examples that suggest that our healthcare system
could indeed be better than the current one and cost less.

Largely unnoticed within the mainstream system of healthcare
today lie a range of diverse perspectives and cultural anomalies
that don't fit the prevailing story. Within a dynamic complex
system such as healthcare there are bound to be counter-trends
and dissenting voices, but they remain marginalised and invisible
to the current mainstream. Yet the fact remains that if we
imagine a more viable future healthcare system we will then
certainly be able to find elements of what we desire hidden in
plain sight within current practice. Another pattern then comes
into view — the patterning of hope.

So what should we look for? Much of this book has stressed
the importance of seeing healthcare as a culture, a set of
assumptions, practices and beliefs not simply a technical service.
We also understand disease as more than a function of individual

biomechanics and itself a reflection of the way we live our lives —
in a late modern culture under strain.

It should come as no surprise then to hear that what we
need to seek out is evidence of a shift in culture — such that
healthcare is once again understood as a living, human system.
This is a qualitative shift in understanding beyond healthcare as
a mechanical and industrial process. This chapter begins with a
description of the South Central Foundation (SCF) healthcare
system in Alaska — a remarkable, large-scale example of this
principle lived out in practice. I have had the privilege of visiting
SCF twice and also welcoming some of its founding practitioners
and its inspirational Chief Executive, Katherine Gottlieb, to
Scotland. It is my contact with SCF that has restored my faith in
healthcare and convinced me that another future is possible. It
is all and more than I could have imagined and is what led me to
write this book.

But SCF is not alone. Perhaps once you have seen and
experienced such a rich alternative so evidently based in a
paradigm of wholeness and humanity it becomes easier to
recognise its pattern and its features in other places. Certainly
I now see elements of the Alaskan approach everywhere. In
Scotland I have worked in recent years to reveal, support and
connect this pattern where I see it, to introduce projects and
programmes and approaches consistent with it where I can, and
consciously to shift my own practice to match its underlying
philosophy. This is an approach to change that is less about
shifting the entire system on to a new footing and more about
quietly revealing and supporting the growth of the new system
that already lies within.

This chapter starts with the SCF story and then expands on
significant elements of the approach that I believe are critical,
that can be replicated and are already evident in diverse practice
elsewhere. The final chapters of the book will explore how to
grow this practice such that it can eventually fulfil its potential to

deliver a healthcare system that is sustainable, contains costs and restores effectiveness.

South Central Foundation, Alaska

The story starts in the 1980s when the Alaskan Native community had grown frustrated at the poor quality of education and healthcare available to it through the US federal government. As part of the settlement that ceded the State of Alaska to the USA, the native community was guaranteed free education and healthcare, but the quality was very poor. Within the healthcare system, everyone was frustrated. Patients had to wait for everything — visits to Accident and Emergency, out-patient departments, the pharmacy, etc. Staff were also frustrated as there seemed to be no end to demand. Population health measures were some of the worst in the USA. And the cost of the service kept rising.

As part of the wider international movement to recognise indigenous rights, the Alaskan Native community took it upon themselves to negotiate with the federal government to take over the running of the health service itself. In 1992 the US government eventually agreed, on condition that this did not lead to requests for increases in funding. Realising that nothing short of a radical reform would both improve services and control costs, South Central Foundation, one of a number of Alaskan Native healthcare providers, undertook a two-year community listening process to find out what the people really wanted from their health service and how they wanted to be treated. Then they delivered it.

The result is a health system where families and communities have taken ownership of their own wellness and recovery. SCF uses an Alaskan Native word 'Nuka' to describe their model. The word means a "strong, large, living structure". The mission of the organisation is to work together with the Native Community to achieve wellness through health and related services. Its vision is a Native Community that enjoys physical, mental, emotional and spiritual wellness. Patients are called customer-owners to reflect the fact that they are no longer passive recipients of care. Instead, they have an active stake in making decisions about their health and how their healthcare is provided. Its approach is based on quality relationships between the healthcare provider and the community it serves, between individual clinicians and patients and between staff so that they work in a seamless and integrated way. They are committed to sharing responsibility for health between their customer-owners and providers, demonstrating quality and promoting family wellness.

Between 1997 and 2007, the results have been remarkable — a reduction of more than 40% in A&E usage, a 50% drop in referrals to specialists, and a decrease in primary care visits by 20%. At the same time, overall health outcomes are better and patient and staff satisfaction is exceptional. In 2012 SCF won the coveted Malcolm Baldrige National Quality Award, the highest level of national recognition for performance excellence that a US public organization can receive. Don Berwick, founder of the Institute of Healthcare Improvement (IHI), has described Nuka as the future not only for US healthcare but for healthcare around the world — and there is now growing international interest.

The Nuka approach has delivered improvements in cost and quality and in reduced demand for services — which has proved a powerful advertisement. Yet SCF did not set out with the intention of shifting those numbers. They instead designed a system consonant with their values, owned by the Alaskan Native people and always responsive to their wishes — and then had the courage to put that into practice. By placing their values and commitment in the foreground the issues this book has been describing have been effectively addressed almost as a side effect. It is an astonishing story.

Intentional design

SCF describes the transformation of the healthcare system as a result of "intentional design". It started small and gradually took over more elements of the health service. When the need arose to build a new primary care centre this too was designed intentionally, in line with its shared values. They know that healthcare environments have to look well. South Central Foundation has won awards for its buildings. They are inspired by Alaskan Native designs, use local materials and are light and airy places. At the front entrance of the hospital is a circular gathering place with comfortable seating and light coming in from the roof. It encourages people to sit and chat and is well used by the local community — whether they are visiting for treatment or not — particularly in the cold winter months.

Similar qualities are seen in the UK in Maggie's Centres, which are cancer information and drop-in centres designed by leading architects. In their book *The Architecture of Hope,* Charles Jencks and Edwin Heathcote describe how each Maggie's Centre is unique but has three features in common: a feeling of homeliness, centred around a kitchen table; widespread use of art works; and a calm, almost sacred feel[50]. These qualities derive from an understanding of the needs of their visitors as well as referring back to the old concept of a 'hospital'. In the Middle Ages hospitals were part of monasteries where the poor, the sick and pilgrims were taken care of. The root in Latin is *hospes,* which means either guest or host, suggesting a mutuality in the encounter — both are giving and receiving.

More mundanely, SCF also pay attention to the way spaces implicitly configure the kinds of interactions and conversations that can comfortably take place in them. Since staff work in highly integrated teams, office space is non-heirarchical — the doctor, nurses and receptionist for each team work in the same room with same-sized desks. The consultation room is called a 'talking room' because 80% of primary care visits only require a conversation and very simple examinations. The room has equal-sized chairs and both doctor and patient sit the same side of the computer. Adjacent to the talking room is a more conventional examination space, should this be required.

Much consultation work is undertaken by phone, which patients are happy with because they know also that SCF guarantees same day access to a healthcare provider if necessary. If you need a face-to-face interview, this can be for anything between ten and forty minutes. Whilst you make your way to the primary care centre, your records are reviewed so that any other check-ups or screening tests are carried out at the same time. This saves multiple visits which push up costs for providers and patients.

A further variation in the design of SCF is the use of family rooms. These can hold up to fifteen people and have a speaker phone to allow more distant relatives to be part of a consultation. The purpose of these rooms is to make sure everyone who is involved in the care and support of the sick person is aware of the diagnosis, prognosis and what can be expected in terms of management. For example, if an older person is diagnosed with dementia, the whole family can be briefed about the implications and preparations made to deal with the inevitable decline. For all our talk of 'integration' and 'joined up' services, it is very rare to find this simple commitment to bringing the human system of care into view in our own system, even while technology has made it so simple in practice.

Health, ownership and autonomy

There are many aspects of the SCF philosophy and practice that hark back to another famous example of intentional design for health - the Pioneer Health Centre in Peckham. Back in the 1920s a pair of doctors in South London broke ranks with their peers in deciding to discover the enabling conditions that might lead to health rather than the patterns of disease. They found that the key to good health was family and relationship: it was impossible to be healthy alone. As a result they decided to create a centre for families, deliberately designed to cultivate the conditions for good health. The Pioneer Health Centre in Peckham opened in 1930 as an airy, spacious place with lots of natural light. There was a swimming pool and gym, a café, two crèches — one for infants, another for toddlers - and a large activity room which had a stage and space for dancing. Families would pay a weekly subscription to use the centre any time from two o'clock in the afternoon to ten o'clock at night. At its height there were over 700 families visiting each day, roughly 1600 people.

Today such a centre would probably be known as a Healthy Living Centre. Examples include the Bromley-by-Bow Health Centre in East London and the Bunnyhill Health Centre in Sunderland. But where the Peckham Experiment differed was in the ownership of the centre by its members and the self-organisation of activities. There were very few rules. People were able to set up activities around whatever interests they had, provided no-one else in the centre was excluded from participating. Children were free to use any of the equipment so long as they put it back in its place afterwards. There were no coaches, trainers or designated life-guards. Safety was maintained by people looking out for each other. The design of the space opened up a wide range of experiences for people to try out and everyone could choose what to do when it suited them. The Pioneer Health Centre was a curated space, designed to create the conditions for health. It was not just the building, but the way in which it was used that generated a sense of health and wellbeing for the people using it.

The Centre collected data on family health but sadly many of the records were destroyed by fire so it is not possible to point specifically to evidence for its health-giving properties. However, in a series of books about the project there are many fascinating stories and anecdotes about its impact on children and adults alike. Several former members when asked what the Centre's greatest single benefit was to them reported having access to a doctor who was also a friend; the freedom to do what you liked when you liked; the long-term friendships they made; the confidence it gave them; the fact it was a family club — a place where all the family liked to go. Families tended to become more united as individual members blossomed in the environment. One of the founding doctors, Innes Pearse, explained how children grow like plants — you cannot cause a plant to absorb nutrients from the soil, but you can tend to the quality of that soil. The focus for parents therefore shifted from what they would give to their children to modeling it in their own lives by being active, engaged and learning new skills. "It is only by their own development, physical and mental, that they can enrich the home, and it is the home ultimately which is the child's environment. This is the soil in which the human seedling must grow." [51]

Many of Peckham's underlying principles are now becoming understood as prerequisites for good health — quality relationships, attention to maternal health from the moment when a couple consider starting a family, wholesome, fresh, locally grown food, physical activity, family wellness and social gatherings. The doctors saw health as being the flow of life through many forms. Life is fundamentally whole, each person and family is a whole within a whole, each with a propensity for growth and development, given the right conditions.

Despite its local popularity (it re-opened after the war due to popular demand), the Centre did not survive the creation of the NHS in 1948. Its emphases on health rather than disease, family rather than individual, community ownership rather than state or independent contractors, were not in keeping with the times.

Salutogenesis — restoring a sense of coherence and manageability in people's lives

Current systems of healthcare are focused on fixing people when they are ill, detecting diseases before they become a problem and telling people to change their self-harming behaviours. As previous chapters have explained, these strategies have limited effectiveness in the face of contemporary patterns of 'dis-ease'.

A different approach is derived from a theory of 'salutogenesis' described by Antonovsky who studied survivors of the Holocaust. He was interested in what helped survivors to defy expectations and live to a ripe old age. Antonovsky found that people who could frame their suffering in ways that made sense to them were able to manage their lives better and live longer as a result.

Restoring meaning and purpose is a vital part of preventing ill health and promoting recovery. The traditional disease prevention metaphor has a fence put up to stop people falling into the river where they would otherwise need to be rescued. In contrast, Antonovsky describes a river of life, where everyone is swimming. In this metaphor, disease is not something that can be prevented as such, but a possibility to be navigated in the rapids and eddies which form part of the river. Some people are good swimmers and can manage these twists and turns easily. Others are less confident and need to take refuge on a rock or hold on to others to stop themselves drowning.

This metaphor helps shape a different pattern of healthcare: rather than stopping people getting into the river or rescuing them when they find they can't swim, it aims to help them swim. Rather than telling them what to do from the banks, staff are also in the river, showing how it's done.

Most of modern healthcare has been built around 'pathogenesis'. It has been great at fixing worn-out parts, treating infections, supplementing low levels of hormones and re-canalising blocked arteries. But there are also some areas where the model is more one of 'salutogenesis', where people are helped to restore coherence in their lives restoring meaning, purpose and a feeling of wellness.

For example, within mental health and addiction services, there is a growing enthusiasm for a 'recovery' approach. Whilst medication is useful in the acute stages of mental illness, longer term recovery requires that people find their own narrative for why they became unwell and create an outlet to discover a deeper meaning and value in their lives. People have found music, art, poetry, journaling, wilderness treks, gardening and all kinds of craft activities useful in re-discovering and re-inventing a sense of themselves[52].

Increasingly people in recovery are becoming peer workers and supports for others who are at an earlier stage in their recovery journey. The act of helping someone else as a way of paying back for help previously received can be a deeply rewarding and therapeutic experience in its own right. Equally, receiving care and treatment from someone who is on their own journey of recovery is comforting. You can sense the future ahead — there is light at the end of the tunnel.

In the small town of Aboyne, ten miles west of Aberdeen, a small project helps injured soldiers recover with help from horses. Jock, an ex-marine, and his wife Emma grew up with horses and over a two week course teach war veterans to become familiar with the animals and eventually ride them, cowboy-style. Horseback UK has attracted attention for its whole-person approach to recovery. The horses do not see the soldier's deformities. As the soldiers learn to communicate with and look after the horses, they recover a sense of self-worth. Riding a horse also raises you above ground level so you can feel seen

and valued. For many of the veterans the highlight of their time
is riding in front of their families. In the space of two weeks
they move from wounded ex-soldier to cowboy. Recovery is not
simply about function and the activities of daily living, but about
personhood, identity, self-worth. So often in current healthcare
the focus and attention is on functional improvement, which
overlooks the existential need for value and purpose in life
particularly in the face of the catastrophic loss of a limb, sight or
hearing. Occupational Therapy students are now learning about
rehabilitation and recovery through attachments to Horseback
UK.

   There is a resonance between this example and the work of
Ludwig Guttman during and following the Second World War.
Guttmann fundamentally disagreed with the medical view at that
time that people with paraplegia were likely to die in weeks or
months. When Guttmann arrived at Stoke Mandeville Hospital
soldiers from the battle front who had broken backs and were
suffering from paraplegia were delivered in coffins and were sent
to a ward out of sight of other patients. Guttmann refused to let
this continue. He would not give up on his fellow human beings
in this way.

   He first changed the way the men were treated — he had them
moved regularly to avoid the build up of pressure sores and the
possibility of urinary tract infections. Then he started to engage
them in physical and skill-based activities. Sports like archery
improved their mental wellbeing while learning new skills, such
as woodwork, clock and watch repair and typing, would ensure
they would be employable when they left hospital. Guttmann
then had the idea of introducing sporting competitions
between staff and patients and with other hospitals. The Stoke
Mandeville Games began on the same day as the 1948 Olympics
in London. When the games went to Rome in 1960 they became
the Paralympics. People who have experienced devastating
loss through trauma or by birth can now show us through their
remarkable performances at these games the extraordinary

potential of human beings given the right environment of encouragement and support.

Quality relationships, quality conversations

SCF operates from an underlying insight that good quality relationships produce better health and underpin effective healthcare. The foundation of quality relationships is an ability to tell our own personal story and listen to those of others.

Because the Nuka model is based on quality human relationships, trust builds between patients, their families, staff and the wider community. Patients and their families are known to the primary care teams, who look after them. Every health encounter is seen first as a conversation and second as a diagnostic and treatment process. As they say, "people have diseases, diseases don't have people".

Similar changes in conversations are taking place in the UK. At their heart is an understanding that for chronic, complex conditions, patients must be in control, be offered meaningful choices and be able to relate to their care providers as partners in care. This has lots of advantages over current systems. Normal clinical practice focuses on specific diseases, creating pathways of care that run in parallel, aiming to control symptoms separately for different conditions. Another way is to ask what patients really want in their lives and configure resources around those goals. It turns out that this autonomy also makes available people's own resources for self-healing and living well with untreatable conditions.

A cardiologist in the North West of England, for example, has developed this approach for people who have severe and complex angina and whose coronary arteries are narrowed in so many different places that stents, re-vascularisation or other forms of surgery would be high risk and offer little prospect of meaningful gain. Instead, he offers to help them without surgery or other major interventions to achieve what they hope for in the remainder of their lives.

Take Joe who was 74 with long-standing high blood pressure who had already had two heart attacks and a prior bypass and was limited to walking 100 metres because of his intractable angina. His one wish was to go to Canada to see his granddaughter. His original cardiologist refused to say he was fit to fly unless he underwent a risky repeat bypass procedure, which he did not want. The patient-centred cardiologist agreed to work with the family to achieve his objectives. The solution was for the patient to pay for his granddaughter to fly to England to visit him. This avoided the unnecessary risk and cost of a redo bypass. Having meaningful goals in life is what makes it worth living. People can manage with a great deal of pain and disability if they have an incentive to keep going. Whilst not their main purpose, conversations of this type also tend to avoid futile investigations and treatment and thus save money.

In Fife, Scotland, occupational therapists, physiotherapists and nurses have changed how they assess older people using conversations focused on personal outcomes. This opens up a different way of understanding how they might regain and maintain mobility and the capacity to look after themselves. Rather than being content merely to ensure their safety and that they are managing to undertake the routine activities of daily living, staff explore with older people what would help them thrive. The results are often very simple but powerful because they are what the older people have chosen for themselves. For Mary with Parkinson's disease it was being able to serve tea in china cups from a trolley for her friends instead of being provided with a safe-pour plastic beaker for her tea and sitting in her kitchen making it by herself. For Joan who had mobility problems, it was walking to the shops, not so that she could buy groceries (it was possible to deliver these) but so that she could chat to her friends and neighbours along the way. Working to achieve these outcomes is highly motivating for the patients and deeply satisfying for the staff. Giving patients autonomy in this way lifts their mood and sustains them in their homes for longer[53].

A similar project in NHS Kernow in Cornwall where volunteers rather than healthcare practitioners undertake these conversations with older people has demonstrated reductions in unplanned admissions to hospital, reduced costs and fewer referrals to social services[54]. These kinds of simple, human solutions have the potential to reduce demand on health systems in the longer term.

Development and growth: learning our way to health

Health is not just the absence of disease but something much more dynamic. Healthy people have a positive sense of vitality; they feel truly alive, and live in connection with others and the world. In other words, when healthy, we are living in equilibrium, giving and receiving warmth and attention to and with each other. The energy and information flowing through and between us are in balance, we feel calm and coherent. Life makes sense. When we fall into negative patterns of life such as over-eating, or misusing alcohol or become depressed, we lose our equilibrium. Our relationships with other people and our environment become distorted. Aside from physical pain that might be part of our condition, we experience a disjunction with the world around us, which is stressful and alienating. We are out of sorts and our world can shrink into focusing on one day, one hour, surviving, not thriving. We feel alone. Without help, this dissonance can start to erode our self-belief: life loses meaning.

Becoming well in this context is about restoring connection with life — through a healthy relationship with ourselves, other people and the wider world. This means taking care of ourselves and what we eat, having enough rest and working on the quality of our relationships. It also requires us to search for and find a sense

of meaning and purpose in our lives[55]. This is a developmental task. In the words of C.G. Jung, "We don't solve our problems, we outgrow them".

Based on this insight, Wellness Enhanced Learning (WEL) classes have been set up by a GP in Nairn, Scotland for her patients with chronic conditions and for staff in the practice. Devised and supported by Dr David Reilly, the originator of the programme, the GP provides a two-hour session to each cohort every Monday afternoon for a month[56].

The main purpose of WEL is to sow ideas and practices that foster self-care, self-compassion and ultimately, healing change. The therapeutic environment is consciously designed to be a welcoming space: one that is 'alive' and where participants can feel safe to express themselves in their own ways. The course includes 'Heart Math' a simple mindfulness technique that puts a person in touch with their inner feelings, their compassion and allows them to become more present in the moment. Using simple metaphors, such as a thriving house plant, participants are invited to describe how they feel and what it would take to help them feel better. So, for example, if they feel they are wilting, in need of water, they think about what this would mean in their lives. It may involve taking things more slowly, spending time in nature or putting aside time to play with their children.

The group learns about diet, being encouraged simply to "eat food"[59]. In practice, this means people reduce their intake of processed foods and cook more from scratch. The programme is not health education in its traditional sense, rather learning how to notice and feed life so that it flows more effortlessly.

Whilst the outcomes of this work are still in the process of evaluation, the signs are encouraging. Patients are managing chronic pain and diabetes more successfully, staff are feeling more positive at work. Participants also notice how much the quality of their family life has improved. They have learned to listen more carefully which has led to greater understanding of children and spouses.

The WEL programme is but one example of a new practice of integrative medicine that aims to bring together the best from traditional and non-traditional approaches to health and healing. US cardiologist Dean Ornish has used these approaches in treating people with heart disease. He has shown that a programme combining lifestyle changes and attention to the underlying reasons for damaging behaviours, including lack of love and intimacy, can reverse the disease process and in many cases lead to the avoidance of surgery. Ornish has more than forty insurance companies funding his programme because it makes such good business sense[58].

Improve healthcare systemically

Because SCF sees itself as a "large, living structure", it is looking to support growth — in people and in learning as a system. It uses improvement methods extensively to understand its performance and to enhance it. GPs record the level of control in blood sugar for their diabetic patients, for example. Those with outstanding results are visited and asked how they have achieved this and whether they would be willing to share their success with others. The emphasis of the organisation is to strive for excellence as a whole system, not penalise poor performers.

The people at SCF don't say, we are "world-class", "excellent" or the "best in class". Rather they say, "we've come a long way, but there is much more we could learn and want to do". In other words, SCF is interested in development, asking not whether it is the best, but if it could be better. Its view of 'better' goes way beyond the 'pit-stop' ideas of excellence — faster, leaner, cleaner — because it believes anything is possible. Its culture is one of openness to the future, whilst staying true to its values. It is quick to learn from the best around the world, but sticks to its core values of shared responsibility, commitment to quality and family wellness when introducing changes. It also tracks the results of its work carefully, using this feedback to shape its next steps. In other words it harnesses the relatively mechanistic and

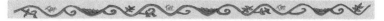

bureaucratic procedure of measuring and calculating, testing and reflecting, not to make single incremental improvements in the status quo but in support of its deeper purpose.

Train people for the job that needs doing

SCF invests in its people as seriously as it invests in its buildings, offering a wide range of training and development opportunities. It tries as far as possible to remove barriers to career progression. The Chief Executive started out as a receptionist in the organisation. Many doctors were previously nurses. It sees skills development as the easy part. But it has to recruit people with the right attitude — one that puts the patient in the driving seat, is willing to work as part of an integrated team and is ready to innovate, striving always for learning and improvement.

In Uganda high school graduates have been trained to become assistants to eye surgeons. After one year they can assess patients and carry out simple procedures. With further training they become cataract surgeons. Their complication rates are no worse than those of qualified doctors who undertake this work. In Mozambique carefully selected community health workers are trained to do obstetric surgery and have been highly successful in improving access to this vital service[57]. Dental health aides operate in a number of rural areas around the world to undertake simple dental procedures. A two-year training programme followed by on-the-job supervision enables them to carry out tooth extraction as safely as fully trained dentists.

These examples point to the potential for life-saving yet simple medical techniques to be carried out by people trained specifically to do them. By contrast, training regimes in the UK require an ever greater range of skills and competencies to be achieved to get admitted on to courses, to qualify and to progress in specialist training. Most doctors are still taking exams into their mid-thirties. Might these more pragmatic approaches yet have a place to play in our own more 'developed' healthcare systems?

Use evidence in context

Evidence derived from randomised controlled trials and other quantitative methods has to be interpreted with caution in practice. But it is possible to get the best of both worlds — led by evidence from trials but supported by experience from practice.

At a pain clinic in Oxford, England, doctors know that there will be significant numbers of patients started on pain killers who will see no benefit from them.

Like all of us, they know that studies report on *average* reductions in pain and not on each patient individually. Unlike most of us, these doctors are treating that knowledge seriously. They stop drugs for patients who have had no relief using them and try a different one *of the same class* before they try different classes of drugs and other treatments[60].

In effect, these doctors are translating evidence from n=x number of patients to n=1, the individual patient seeking help. Whilst using the evidence of efficacy from drug trials, they use an empirical approach with each person recognising that everyone responds in their own particular way. Yet in doing so they are having to fight the system.

Clinical guidance is based on average effects and so it tends to restrict the range of treatment options. Usually only one or two drugs in the same class are recommended before adding drugs of different classes and other treatments into the mix. The effect is to escalate the number and types of drugs given with a significant proportion of people taking them for no individual benefit. The doctors in Oxford suggest that less restrictive guidance which is centred on the patient-clinician interaction and "a large dose of clinical wisdom" as well as evidence would be better.

Another way of describing this is that doctors need to be both captains and pilots. Doctors can use evidence-based guidance as the captain of a vessel will use navigational charts to head to port. But when coming in to dock, the captain welcomes on board a pilot, someone who knows the nuances of the local river, its particular hazards and landmarks. In selecting the path for a patient, knowledge of the evidence from trials helps to determine a range of options for treatment, but it is also essential to know and understand their patients' unique circumstances, their aspirations and their individual responses to treatment.

Real-time communication for service integration and patient empowerment

Supporting and enabling both patients and staff to make decisions in the face of uncertainty around diagnosis, treatment and recovery can be a challenge. However, simple methods such as email and text messages can help. For example, a cardiologist in Wales introduced email support to GPs to help them manage patients with heart problems. He guaranteed a response within 48 hours of receiving a query. This simple device reassured GPs that in the majority of cases they were managing patients appropriately so they didn't need to send them up to a clinic. The cardiologist saw a rapid fall in referrals as the GPs found they could handle more of the caseload themselves. Those who did attend the cardiology clinic had highly complex conditions requiring his level of expertise, which was a much better use of his time[63].

In a similar way simply keeping in text contact with patients following discharge from an alcohol detoxification programme can help them feel supported in their ongoing journey of recovery. Services sometimes fear providing open access to patients in this way, but they rarely abuse the trust they have been given and use the method of communicating only when they need to. Results from a small study in Bolton showed a significant reduction in re-referrals for detox services in patients receiving these text messages, saving their service an estimated £100,000 per year[64].

Similar use of simple telecommunications comes from London where young people attend their diabetic clinic via Skype video on their mobile phones. This project has demonstrated improved satisfaction with the service and better diabetic control[61]. With better control, there are fewer complications such as hospital admissions due to diabetic ketoacidosis.

Telemedicine and telecare solutions are growing by the day, but need to be viewed with some caution. Where they are part of an enabling, humanising culture, which seeks to enhance human interaction to build quality relationships, they can be very supportive. But put into a distant culture of surveillance, these solutions can reduce human interaction and create greater alienation between patients and their care providers. The examples given above were successful because they used existing technologies for healthcare purposes rather than inventing new ones, effectively bringing healthcare closer to people's everyday lives. Each supported greater interaction between different people in the system, often responding in real- or close to real-time, and facilitated two-way communication. They were part of a healthcare culture that sees the value in enhancing human relationships.

Help patients and staff to share their stories

One of SCF's core programmes is the Family Wellness Warriors Initiative (FWWI) which aims to "eliminate domestic abuse, child abuse and child neglect in the State of Alaska within this generation". At the heart of the FWWI programme is becoming aware of one's own life story and how it has shaped personal beliefs, relationships, attitudes and behaviours. It is community-led, with SCF providing a safe space for people to share their stories at a deep level with each other. This builds trust and repairs relationships that have been damaged. It also grows people's capacity to support others to make the same journey towards wellness.

SCF noticed that people who went through the FWWI programme had a different expectation of their healthcare providers. They were seeking deeper relationships with them and wanted to become more active participants in their care and treatment. As a result they now run a modified version of FWWI for staff working in the organisation. Core Concepts, as the programme is called, helps staff to build trusting relationships with each other, develop good listening skills and share their personal stories in ways that are affirming and respectful. This puts staff at ease with patients and makes them better equipped to encourage patients to take the steps needed to become well, since this is what they too are doing in their own lives. They are all learning to swim better in the river of life.

Around Scotland there is a growing network of Chaplaincy Listeners who spend time in primary care settings simply listening to a patient's story. The Listeners (mainly volunteers, often retired Chaplains and other pastoral workers) are supervised by NHS Chaplains. The pastoral care model that they work to helps patients suffering ill health address existential questions such as: "why me?", "why now?", "what is life about?". The process aims to help patients find meaning, control and confidence in themselves and hope for the future[62].

Whilst in its early stages, feedback from GPs is encouraging. They believe the service eases pressure on other counselling and talking therapies and knowing it is there as an option provides comfort and support for them as well as for patients. Recognising that these patients needed to look at their lives, rather than be given pills, GPs believe their own prescribing has become more effective as a result.

It is not uncommon for clinical situations to raise emotional and ethical issues for staff, yet they rarely get the chance to discuss such things. Values-based Reflective Practice is being developed in Scotland to help healthcare professionals share difficult stories from practice and receive feedback from their peers in a safe and non-blaming way. Using phrases like, "I notice that..." or "I am wondering if..." professionals can receive constructive comments about their practice. In addition, they are asked "Whose needs are being met in the situation you were describing?" which helps health staff separate out their own needs from those of the patients they are caring for.

This practice is enabling healthcare professionals to become more reflective practitioners which in turn helps them make difficult decisions, clear in the knowledge they are being made in the interests of the patient and not themselves. In one discussion Dr Alex came to see how she put Mrs Jones, a patient with long-standing and advanced-stage heart failure, onto renal dialysis because she felt under pressure at the time to do something. On reflection, Dr Alex was able to see that Mrs Jones was dying and further invasive treatment was not in her interest. Understanding the human dynamics involved in patient care could lead to far better use of high-tech interventions and, whilst not its main purpose, would reduce healthcare costs.

Developing reflective practice in this way effectively offers an alternative approach to quality in healthcare. As Ballat and Campling have pointed out in their book *Intelligent Kindness,* rather than cajoling and chasing poor practice, an alternative would be to support and enable staff to do what they want to do in most cases — provide great care[65]. In setting up the Center for Professionalism and Peer Support, Harvard Medical School is realising the importance of this. It now provides one-to-one peer support for any clinician who is involved in an 'adverse event' so that they are able to process its emotional impact and learn lessons for the future. This is now valued as such an important part of care that being a clinician mentor counts for promotion in the organisation in the same way as publishing peer-reviewed research papers.

Taking time to reflect, share stories and develop skills for self-care and mindfulness can help healthcare staff be more confident and resilient in the face of the emotional demands of the job. With this in mind, healthcare staff in Ayrshire have been using a practical resource called Kitbag in team meetings and individually[66]. Many have taken it home to use with their families. Inspired by the ideas in Kitbag, staff are now developing an onsite wellness centre for staff along the lines of the Oasis centres in Hong Kong set up after the SARS epidemic claimed many healthcare staff amongst its victims.

Governance and ownership: citizen-led healthcare

Part of the attraction of the spaces created at SCF is the sense of ownership they encourage. The governance of SCF is also important. SCF is managed by a Board of Governors, all Alaskan Natives, from different tribes in the region. They are a group of wise elders who were prepared to take over and run their own healthcare system. Funding comes from the federal government in a block grant. Other income comes from Medicare and other health insurance where customer-owners are eligible. The Board knew they were taking on a huge challenge. The previous system was broken. It would take time to grow a new one, based on Alaskan Native values. Bringing the community with them was crucial, hence they undertook a two-year listening exercise and continue with ongoing dialogue to ensure the system is always shaped by the needs of their customer-owners.

Most debates about healthcare reform in the UK tend to polarise between public or private ownership. There are few examples of community-owned healthcare systems. In the past, many towns built hospitals by public subscription and these were run by charities. There is often loyalty to hospitals built in this way but little recognition of the value of this approach in encouraging ownership of healthcare more widely by local people. GPs in the UK can be salaried employees or independent contractors within the NHS, but the governance of primary care is poorly developed. A few general practices have become social enterprises, others have extensive partnerships with local agencies to create healthier options for their patients, but being accountable to patients who form a Board of Directors for the practice is virtually unheard of.

The reason why ownership is important to SCF is because it places the control of health and healthcare with the people themselves. They are offered options and are free to make their own decisions. In target and protocol-driven systems, this can be difficult, particularly if income is dependent on adhering to their demands. This shift in control represents an act of faith — trusting that people know what is best for them and can make decisions about their health accordingly. This may be against medical advice at one point, but at another the person can change their mind and come back for treatment.

Clearly there are limits to this approach. Where someone is badly injured, unconscious even, they need urgent medical attention and control shifts towards clinicians. However, the overall aim is to let go of that control as the patient recovers to the point where they are fully in command of decisions about their health when they enter longer term recovery and rehabilitation or when they experience chronic or life-changing conditions.

SCF recognises that patients and staff need help with this change in power and control. Within its primary care teams it has 'behavioural health consultants' (BHCs), trained psychologists, who aim to support patients to take charge of their own health. In addition to helping patients address their health concerns, the BHC offers support and guidance to other members of the primary care team. SCF recognises that everyone working in healthcare has their own healing journey to make. BHCs support staff in this process, particularly when difficult emotional issues arise — sometimes because of what is happening with patients, sometimes because of team dynamics. Having emotional support available on demand is important in maintaining the long term motivation and commitment of staff.

Facing death

So long as there is a flicker of life, it can be the generator of more life — even in the face of death. Indeed, where death seems inevitable, life has its greatest opportunity for expression. This has been written about poignantly by Victor Frankl, who survived Auschwitz[67]. In this most extreme place, those who lost a reason to live would die within two weeks — usually falling ill with typhus or some other infection. Despair kills. However, even those on their way to the gas chambers were able to give life. Frankl recalls being given a tiny folded copy of a prayer from the Talmud by someone in the death queue. The act left Frankl feeling a profound sense of gratitude and love and helped him to keep going, knowing he was part of a wider community. Hope is the experience of life in death. It is deeply restoring.

In traditional cultures, death is seen as a sacred and mysterious journey into the spirit world. At SCF, family and friends of a loved one will be with the dying person for days, often singing, dancing, praying and using their traditional healing practices of burning sage and giving massage. They are particularly appreciative of the role of elders during these difficult times even if they do nothing more than sit with the dying person for a few hours. They see this as the elder, "gracing us with their presence". When the time for words is over, there is still the chance simply to be, which offers comfort and support.

Modern society does not have a vibrant myth about death, which can make it more difficult for us to face. But one of the great privileges in providing healthcare is to offer support and compassion to others who are facing their last journey. The lesson from SCF is that it need not involve anything more than sitting with the dying patient and their loved ones.

Having a clinician who has hope for you and your future,
even in the face of death, is a great comfort. In most healthcare
situations today, being a partner is more important than being a
hero. This is surely the critical area in which the rhetoric about
patient choice will now be put to its most difficult and delicate
test. In a 'healthcare as product and patient as consumer'
paradigm, patient choice can mean little more than being able
to decide which hospital to go to for an operation. Yet what is
more meaningful for patients, and what many are now asking
for, are real choices about how they manage their condition.
It takes courage on the part of our clinicians to open up these
conversations, but when the options on offer are genuine,
patients can be truly empowered to make their own decisions
about their care.

In many kidney units, medical teams are offering people
with end-stage kidney failure a choice of dialysis treatment or
no dialysis but home-based nursing support for their condition.
Dialysis treatment is a physical and psychological burden because
patients are attached to a dialysis machine for several hours three
times or more each week or have fluid exchange in and out of
the abdomen each night. An alternative is home-based nursing
support with regular visits from a renal nurse who can address the
side effects of renal failure and provide support and advice leading
to good end-of-life care when that time comes. Studies have
shown that people aged 75 or over with other significant medical
problems such as heart disease or diabetes have a life expectancy
of 15-21 months with conservative treatment and 18-24 months
with dialysis. In other words, for a 3 month reduction in survival,
the quality of life is hugely enhanced and many patients choose
this option. In today's system of healthcare, few people get the
chance to make such choices.

It takes honest, open and realistic conversations with patients
and their families to be able to offer choices such as these.

Paradoxically, some of these options need to be re-invented because technology has become so successful in saving lives. It is all too easy to opt for the latest cancer drug or technical development in the belief that it must be 'better than doing nothing'. It is interesting to note that when doctors themselves are faced with end-of-life decisions they often prefer more conservative options than those they usually advocate for their patients[66]. It seems that we need a rebalancing of care and treatment to include discussion of conservative options when people are perhaps ready to die and do not want to consider further active treatment of their medical problems. This is not the same as assisted suicide or euthanasia, but simply using the medical technology available to us in a wise, responsible and compassionate way.

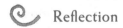 Reflection

The very structure of healthcare undergoes something of a metamorphosis when a recovery and relationship model takes precedence in the management of chronic and complex conditions. Rather than people having to fit the structure of the healthcare system — visiting many different departments for investigation and treatment — support for recovery is brokered and facilitated by healthcare providers in conjunction with a wide variety of other local organisations and support groups. The organisational structure forms around the strength and value of different relationships. The quality of healthcare is not just measured in terms of the skill and expertise of professionals in the system, but the vibrancy of connection between healthcare providers and the resources of their local community.

The examples described above have many lessons for future health systems. First of all, medical pioneers are likely to be regarded with incredulity in their early days. "Where is the

evidence?" people ask, without realising the layers of cultural and conceptual assumptions in the question. Second, a more effective health service can only be built around fresh understandings of what it means to be healthy and resilient. This is not about being either healthy or sick, but being part of a bigger life-death-life process, which is dynamic, relational and cultural. Third, restoring meaning and purpose provides a fundamental drive towards recovery. We all need something to get out of bed for in the morning. In a metaphorical sense, meaning and purpose are like vitamins and their lack curtails life and flourishing. Meaning and purpose cannot be achieved alone but are built with the hope and belief of others.

The combined efforts of people in their own communities offering mutual and reciprocal support to one another, supported by an enabling healthcare infrastructure, offers a new frame for health systems. Rather than configuring all health services around deficits and illness, this frame grows an economy of wellbeing, configuring recovery and aspiration through quality relationships.

CHAPTER 8

Designing for Transition

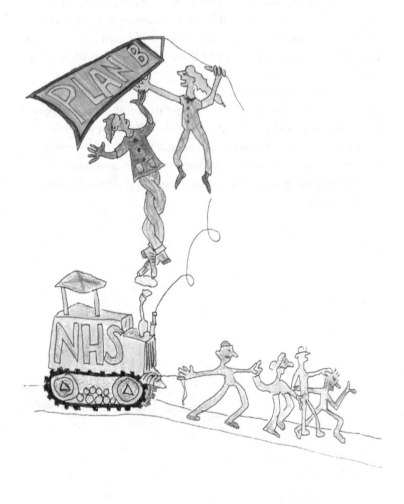

"Gentlemen, we have run out of money. It is time to start thinking."

Sir Ernest Rutherford

Ten years to transform healthcare

As the examples in the last chapter demonstrate, another healthcare system is possible — and is beginning to take shape before our eyes. The new is growing in our midst, even as most of our attention is drawn to the challenges and crises of the old.

In the next chapter I outline a programme — based on my own experience — for how we can all contribute to this transition. But these individual efforts will be much more effective if there is also in place a supportive policy framework, which is what this chapter is about — one that understands the need consciously to design for transition from our existing healthcare system to something very different over the next decade.

From what I have experienced and researched in recent years I am convinced that such a transition is not only necessary but eminently possible. With the right support structures in place, in ten years we can shift the culture to deliver better healthcare than the current system does for the same cost in real terms at worst, and for a substantial cost reduction at best.

Because the approach is to grow what is already there, working with and releasing the creative energies in the system, this will not be an expensive process of top down re-engineering. I believe the shift can be delivered with an investment of just one hundredth of one percent of the current healthcare budget per year for ten years. For the healthcare system I am most familiar with, in Scotland, that amounts to £1,000,000 a year.

This is a bold claim to make but is backed up by everything that has been said in this book so far. Who will be the first Minister of Health to say, "Yes, let's try it. We really have nothing to lose."?

The case for Plan B

Perhaps the Minister will need a little more detail, beyond the bold promise of transition, in order to be convinced. So what is the story we may need to tell her in order to enroll the power that rests in the current system in support of shaping things for the future. And what — aside from a tiny fraction of the health budget — do we need to ask for?

We can start by recalling the thesis of the early part of this book. Over the last fifty years the world has changed in many ways. The pattern of disease has shifted from acute to chronic and from single diseases to multi-morbidity; there are more patients with dementia and diseases of extreme old age, widening health inequalities as well as increasing obesity-related ill health and more recognition of the impact of trauma in childhood on patterns of adult pathology. Technology has moved on enormously, not just in healthcare but in general, yet healthcare lags behind the public in many ways, particularly in its use of smart phones, tablets and social media. Furthermore, healthcare has also become very much more complex. In the words of Atul Gawande, author of the highly influential *Checklist Manifesto,* "the plane has got too big to fly".

Forecasts about financing our complex healthcare services in the long term are bleak. Either the performance is likely to deteriorate rapidly or an ever-increasing proportion of GDP will be needed to support them. This can only be achieved in real terms by raiding other departmental budgets, pushing the costs directly onto patients, or raising taxes.

Heroic efforts are taking place to keep the current show on the road. Patient safety initiatives, the use of improvement science and the deployment of human factors research help mitigate the impact of falling resources and rising demand on the quality of care — up to a point. But staff wellbeing is suffering. After falls in sickness absence between 2009 and 2012 the trend is now rising again[69]. People are counting the years until retirement or going early. Others are moving to work in parts of the world where economies remain strong, such as Australia or Canada[70]. Recruitment from Africa and the Asian sub-continent is not an ethical option as it leaves impoverished health systems with even fewer skilled workers[71].

We need a Plan B.

The good news is that plenty of people are already working on it. The seeds of a new culture are emerging in the NHS and social care around the UK. Currently this is the work of a few passionate individuals, prepared to go the extra mile with their colleagues and the public. Yet at the same time new policy frameworks are being introduced, for example around chronic disease management, multi-morbidity, total place commissioning, asset-based community development, person-centred care, quality improvement and reablement, which may yet encourage these pioneers to create a real and lasting change of culture.

What is lacking is a connection between these policy frameworks and the reality of healthcare on the ground. Staff are preoccupied with existing pressures and struggle to find time to think or to change their approach. The policy environment itself keeps changing, with politicians responding to the latest scandal around standards of care or missed targets or resource pressures. The media does not help, whipping up public anxiety, searching out scapegoats to blame and excluding nuanced voices calling for a more developmental approach.

With a small investment in catalytic funding — and learning — and a smart policy framework to support it, everything could be very different. It just requires the political will to set in place enabling conditions for the kind of innovation this book advocates rather than implicitly crowding it out in favour of approaches that are more familiar, effective up to a point, necessary but not sufficient and that offer only false hope for the future.

A policy framework for transition

To an extent this is a generic challenge — how to provide a
policy framework for making a transition from one dominant
mode of operation in a large, complex public system to another
over time, while ensuring that operations do not fail in the
process. International Futures Forum call this 'redesigning the
plane whilst flying it', which appears today less like a party trick
and more a core competence for the modern policymaker. The
fullest description of the process is contained in the IFF book
*Transformative Innovation in Education: a playbook for pragmatic
visionaries*. What follows is a version of the policy prescription
for transforming the education system adapted for the special
circumstances of healthcare.

Direction

The first requirement is perhaps the most obvious. We need to
know which direction we want the system to move in. The role
of government is at least to provide a compass direction even
if it cannot supply the map. At the moment our navigation is
more or less explicitly set on providing more of the same at a
more affordable cost. Yet we know that more of the same is not
what we need to address contemporary needs, and that costs
continue to rise even as we try to control them. We are set on a
path to a destination we cannot possibly reach: the first role of
government is to acknowledge that and to legitimise those who
have a different sense of what healthcare could be, even if at this
stage they cannot provide a detailed map of how to get there.

Diversity

Work towards this vision will be led by pioneers and early
adopters within the system. The inevitable, and desirable,
result will be greater diversity of provision. Policy needs to
tolerate, indeed welcome, this variation and be ready with a
response to those who say, "If we cannot do it for everyone, we

should not do it for anyone". Policy will need to become much more sophisticated about how it learns from experiment, how it extracts principles from one place to apply in another and so on. Just as medicine needs to move beyond its reliance on Randomised ControlledTrials and effectiveness based on averages drawn from big numbers, so too policy needs to become more adept at dealing with the unique, the personal, the specific, the set of n=1. And as issues arise that look like choices between mutually exclusive goods — such as universality and diversity — policy needs to practise dilemma thinking in order to get the best of both worlds.

Support

As the previous chapter showed, there is already plenty of activity shifting the healthcare system in a new and more sustainable direction. But it gets little attention, little support and — often — active detraction from dominant systems. Inevitably most of the discourse is about keeping the plane in the air and there is considerable scepticism about the prospects of redesign. Yet for any new system to emerge fully in the future, it will need support from the old. There are a number of ways in which policy can help.

The first is simply to validate and legitimise alternative practice by drawing attention to the quiet efforts of many who are using holistic and relational approaches to address complex, chronic health conditions. Politicians and other health leaders need do no more than seek out and visit places where there are signs of a transformation taking place in terms of relationships, connections with communities and hold out for this as a clear vision of the future. These examples would be like small tiles in a new mosaic of healthcare innovations which, as they grow, will meet needs more effectively in the long term.

A more active contribution is to provide explicit systems of support for those attempting to change culture and practice.

The traditional mode for policy in times of big systems change is to provide instructions and guidance — and then to inspect for achievement and share 'best practice'. The shift I am proposing is too complex, subtle and context-dependent for that. What practitioners need are processes, materials, prompts, advice and experience to help them think through their next moves, their change initiatives, for themselves. IFF, for example, has established a dedicated Practice Centre to provide such resources, not only for healthcare but across the board. A critical role for a central authority like government is then to bring together practitioners into a community for the sake of learning from each other, sharing 'best problems' rather than best practice. This kind of investment in reflective learning for staff is the next 'new build' for healthcare. It should be part of the 21st century capital programme.

Measurement

Government can also help in understanding that evaluation of these efforts will itself require some innovative thinking. Navigating towards an aspirational future in the presence of existing demands is not a linear process in terms of time or steps taken. However, in order to build credibility, recording the journey of transition must be data intensive. The Alaskans have submitted themselves to the most rigorous measurement and evaluation without becoming trapped by it (they say that a model is a shadow of reality, and that data based on any model is therefore a shadow of a shadow of reality). Our own transition efforts should follow the same principle: measuring the things that matter to existing systems at the same time as those that will provide meaningful feedback for local projects in their own terms. In time we will see that these two sets of indicators are linked, but if we privilege the first from the start we will never escape the gravitational pull of existing systems.

Funding

One final area where government can help is in creating more flexible funding arrangements. Tendering exercises require bids to meet preconceived ideas of success whilst pioneers are often working outside these underlying assumptions. Funding calls for innovation often require people to compete with each other whereas working together might generate more synergy and learning in the system. Pioneers may not spend all the funds they are allocated within a set timeframe, but public accounts are constrained from carrying forward funds from one financial year to another. Innovation in funding itself requires careful thought if pioneering activity to grow a new and more effective health system is to succeed.

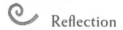 Reflection

Healthcare is not just an industry focused on repairing and replacing worn-out parts. It is human and relational. Restoring its effectiveness in the face of chronic conditions and an ageing population relies on mobilising the creativity and innovation of its participants — staff and patients alike. Policy-makers can set the tone by celebrating people's strengths and resilience, providing opportunities for reflective learning and fostering a culture of trust and transparency.

CHAPTER 9

Creating the Future

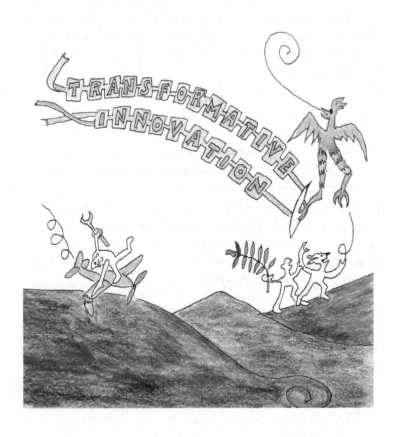

"You never change things by fighting the existing reality. To change something, build a new model that makes the existing model obsolete."

Buckminster Fuller

Start where you are

I am a healthcare practitioner, a doctor who has spent nearly all of her professional life inside the NHS. This book is, therefore, fundamentally empirical — based on my observations of how the system operates in practice and the theoretical and research frameworks that I have been able to draw on over the years to make sense of that experience.

This final chapter will follow the same pattern. I do not propose here a grand theoretical schema for transforming our healthcare systems, a radical policy reform agenda to save the NHS. There are plenty of those available for anyone with the appetite[72]. As I hope I have shown from the start, most of these plans for radical reform are limited by their starting assumptions — cultural assumptions about what counts as evidence, how we conduct 'research', what success looks like and, above all, what we are talking about when we talk about health.

It was Aldous Huxley who said "Medical science has made such tremendous progress that there is hardly a healthy human left". Decades later doctors are beginning to notice that their worldview has the potential for harm[73]. My own journey in medicine has been in search of what makes people healthy and to seek to create the enabling conditions for the natural processes that feed life.

Whether the policy context outlined in the previous chapter is in place or not, we as healthcare practitioners have the opportunity to bring the new system into being in our own work — intervention by intervention, project by project. This chapter tells the story of one such intervention in support of older people

in my local region, and concludes with a short set of guidelines that for me emerge from this and other similar work. I know that these guidelines will ring true to the many practitioners who are already working in this way within the system: for them I hope they will offer support and encouragement. Equally I hope they may inspire others to give this approach a try: we have nothing to lose but our sense of ineffectiveness, frustration and vocation denied.

The Fife Shine story

The 'Shine' initiative — a programme designed to help older people live longer and more fulfilling lives in their own homes and to enable earlier discharge from hospital — has its roots in a growing concern in my local health area, Fife, about how to cope with the demand for emergency admissions. Typically when older people are admitted to hospital, their home circumstances are found to be fragile and so the process of discharging them from hospital and sending them home takes a very long time. This is a national phenomenon and there is in Scotland a coordinated learning process, sharing best practice, that invites every health board to plan annually, particularly for the winter months, and register lessons learned as the spring arrives.

In 2009 one of the lessons learned in Fife was that despite improving on all our systems over the years we were working flat out and could not see ourselves getting through another winter without a significant drop in our performance on waiting times. Resources were already spread too thin. We had reached the conclusion I recorded in Chapter 5: sweating the system harder for greater efficiency was not going to be enough and was already leading to significant collateral damage. We needed to think differently.

That led us to engage in a brief, tightly focused exercise designed to stretch our thinking out beyond incremental improvement to imagine a system that really works and that we would love to work in. We then considered the pathways we might need to explore in order to move from the current system towards our ideal. One of those pathways involved having better, more honest conversations with older people — about the limitations of medical treatment and about their own aspirations for the rest of their lives. This seemed to be part and parcel of what then became a firm commitment which a small team determined to explore in practice: "to help older people thrive, not just survive, in their own homes".

The original team came from public health, community health services and occupational therapy: those parts of the NHS that regularly deal with older people. But over time others became interested in the vision and soon individuals from the local authority were involved, plus people from the voluntary and social enterprise sectors.

We applied for an innovation grant from the Health Foundation under their Shine programme (hence the project name) based on 'invest to save' principles. We suggested that in two years we might be able to close a single continuing care ward through this approach and were given a small grant to get us started.

The essence of the idea was as simple as opening up a 'grown-up' conversation with older people about what matters to them in the rest of their lives and to respond accordingly — supporting their innate capacity for health. The critical shift would therefore need to be a shift in practice, led by those staff — usually the Occupational Therapists — who have the initial conversation with an older person in their own homes. Rather than undertake the normal 'assessment', checking the patient against a pre-existing list of ailments, circumstances and concerns, staff were trained in a simple technique to allow them to get into a real and meaningful conversation.

Older people themselves and their family carers took a while to get used to being asked these questions. They were unused to staff taking the trouble to find out more about their lives in the round. Relatives commented to staff how much they appreciated that someone was now listening. This in itself seemed to lift the mood of older people and helped the staff feel more valued. Above all, the shift in conversation style engaged older people and their families in actively seeking solutions to match the aspirations that had been voiced. The staff began to appreciate the difference between fixing somebody's problems for them and inviting them into a dialogue in which their own inner resources and aspirations become an essential component.

This was not an easy shift to make in practice. Staff had been reluctant to start out on this process, fearing that people would ask for the moon — a request that they would inevitably have to disappoint. But to their surprise they found older people asked for very small things — the chance to get out, to go shopping, to make and serve tea for their friends. With a little resourcefulness and creativity, staff explored with patients how these wishes could be fulfilled — using help from family, neighbours, friends and local small-scale providers.

These were not requests that could be met by existing statutory services. So what emerged was a hidden demand for a very different range of supports. This led the project to start getting involved with, connecting with and growing small-scale services in the community. Local area co-ordinators undertook a mapping of existing activities for older people in communities across Fife and several other projects were catalysed into existence to meet the need that professional staff were beginning to identify. Existing small-scale providers were supported to expand their offer and people with good ideas were encouraged to set up additional activities and services with the help of a local organisation specialising in supporting social enterprise. The project team also undertook the necessary negotiation and design work to ensure that all this new support activity with older people stayed within regulatory requirements. New service providers were given advice on completing disclosure checks, having liability insurance and using the correct transport licence. In short, small-scale providers were supported to become safe, legal and sustainable.

This was slow work. By the end of the first year just five older people had completed a new-style conversation and found a solution to fulfil their wishes. Yet these few stories of success were so simple, so moving and so far removed from what passed for 'service provision' before that all those involved were encouraged to continue. They realised that for this approach to grow as a practice staff would need more support to allow it to become routine. They needed to be confident with the approach and use it with all their patients.

That led to the establishment of peer support groups for the staff to meet monthly to share their stories of working in this way with each other. In these groups they were able to build up their confidence in opening up a different kind of conversation, persist when previously they would have looked for other (often more costly) options and become increasingly inspired by the stories they were hearing. They were discovering hidden resources in themselves, in the older people they were looking after and in the wider community. By the end of the second year, at least fifty older people had experienced a different kind of conversation with staff and found novel ways to meet their aspirations. The work of the social enterprise and voluntary sector side of the project meant that stronger connections with local communities were being made. This uncovered a range of resources which staff were able to access along with informal support from family and friends.

By the close of year two, therefore, the project had demonstrated proof of concept. This approach can work, it does save money and it is possible to scale it beyond a few individual cases. It had not spread fast enough to close a ward as promised — the cultural barriers to introducing such a novel approach in a system already operating at its limits had been considerable. And in practice the ward had been closed in any case in year one, with managers latching on to the existence of the Shine project as cover for finding savings that (as we saw in Chapter 3) had become too urgent to be delayed.

In year three the work was about growing scale and capacity: engaging with others including other services, extending the training to further teams and growing more connections with local communities. From the outset, the pioneers had fostered relationships with social work, the voluntary sector and other parts of the health system. At the policy level in the meantime the direction of travel had been towards advocating closer integration between health and social care, the use of self-directed support (personal budgets) for people accessing social care and a close interest in so-called 'person-centred' approaches. The Shine project came to be seen as an early example of how these aspirations might be achieved at the local level.

Three clinical champions were identified to train more staff and provide them with peer support as they put this training into practice. Older people were invited to coffee mornings to talk about what they would like to see in their local communities to help them live fuller lives. Findings from these conversations were shared with other local people who were looking to make a difference, stimulating greater voluntary initiative in local areas. More small-scale community providers were helped to negotiate hurdles to enable them to become safe, legal and sustainable — extending the diversity and range of options for older people. Some of these hurdles required negotiation with statutory regulators. By the end of the third year, these regulators were also part of the conversation to explore how they too could play a part in realising the aspiration that older people should thrive — not just survive — at home.

After three years, 25 members of staff have been trained in the new approach and are involved in peer support groups, an estimated 1000 older people have had a personal outcome conversation and new solutions found to meet their aspirations. Over 700 older people are accessing small-scale local services either directly from the community or through their conversations with healthcare staff. Older people, their families and friends are noticing the difference — they are saying how they feel human again, they are happier in themselves, more actively engaged in life. Staff too are saying how much they enjoy working in this way. It feels more meaningful and satisfying for them. Interestingly, they say it takes them no extra time to have these conversations compared with the old-style assessments, but they are using their time more intentionally. Building up a relationship with the older person also means it is easier for them to know when they are no longer needed. In some cases, it is the older person who discharges the staff saying with gratitude that their work is done.

Older people are thriving at home using resources that money can't buy. In the economy of wellbeing, money is on the margins not at the centre. It is meaningful conversations that are the currency and mutually satisfying ways to support one another that are the outcome. Small-scale providers offer contributions because they want to: financial compensation is not their main motivation. Whilst there are costs that have to be covered for these new patterns of activity to be sustained, these are small in comparison with the money that can be released in the longer term from decommissioning redundant healthcare infrastructure. A profound culture shift is taking place.

A qualitative improvement methodology

Elements of this story will be familiar to anyone practising the subtle art of innovation in large, complex, over-stressed systems: the need to overcome resistance, to start small and scale, to raise resources from outside the system to get started by promising savings to come. These features are common to most of the improvement methodologies now pressed upon us with ever greater urgency as our healthcare systems falter. One critical difference is that the Shine project was always explicitly a cultural innovation — not simply trying to improve the existing system but to bring about a fundamental shift in the values and assumptions that underpin healthcare practice in this area.

This kind of innovation requires us to pay attention to factors that might otherwise pass un-noticed: people as well as data, the human system of relationships as well as the abstract system of flows and connections, qualities as well as quantities, who we are *being* as much as what we are *doing*. My friends and colleagues in IFF, who have played an important role in supporting the development of the Shine project throughout, call this 'transformative innovation' — shifting the system towards our aspirations rather than just fixing what is failing. Learning from Shine and many other projects with a transformative intent they have over the years begun to formulate a comprehensive 'qualitative improvement methodology'. Its hallmark is engaging all of our human capacities, including creativity and imagination rather than rely on best practice, big data and small tests of incremental improvement.

The following pages draw out from the Shine story the essential phases in such a process.

Take a broader, aspirational view

The Fife Shine project had its origins in a conversation about winter planning. A group of interested parties from across the system concluded that we really needed some new thinking in order to address a growing annual challenge with shrinking resources. IFF invited the group to use a very simple framework around which to build a conversation that would free us up to think beyond the usual boundaries of this conundrum. This is the Three Horizons framework, which invites us to consider three different perspectives on the future, all present (to varying degrees) at any stage in a system's development:

1. The first horizon (H1) represents the dominant system in the present. Since the world is changing, and nothing lasts forever, the H1 perspective on the future is one of challenge and concern and the over-riding interest is in how to maintain the system in the face of present and future threats. Innovation is dedicated to that end — making the system more efficient in order to stave off decline.

2. The third horizon (H3) can be seen as the place where our many different ideal visions for the future cohere and assemble. IFF member Bill Sharpe calls it "the patterning of hope"[74]. As a perspective on the future H3 is visionary and aspirational. Innovation is dedicated to that end — bringing into being aspects of the future we desire, being the change we want to see in the world.

3. Between H1 and H3, the second horizon (H2) is the space where these competing visions collide, a zone of numerous initiatives and innovations. The H2 perspective on the future is one of opportunity — as the world changes so new things become possible. H2 energy is entrepreneurial, keen to try things to see if they work. Innovation is opportunistic in that sense — a thousand flowers blooming.

The diminishing returns on the investment of money and energy suggest that the current way of providing healthcare is an example of H1 under strain. Efforts to keep it propped up through efficiency savings, outsourcing, off-loading care to others by reducing lengths of stay in hospital, may help to maintain it against the grain of changes in the wider world. But nothing lasts forever and if we really want a sustainable healthcare system for the future we need to find ways to renew the current patterns of provision such that they operate in tune with our changing world.

Without a vision of that future sustainable system, all our innovations will inevitably be sucked back into maintaining the first horizon. In the confusing zone of the second horizon, where all kinds of innovation are competing for attention and survival,

the selection mechanisms privilege innovations that will prop up the old system over those that might create the future.

Thus the first requirement, if we want something different, is to articulate our third horizon aspirations. Then we can select transformative innovations which aim to grow a system that is in line with these aspirations. One helpful clue in shaping these innovations is to learn from examples of the third horizon that are already in existence. These may be small scale and, by definition, on the margins of the mainstream but they show us that our aspirations can be fulfilled. This is why learning from SCF is so powerful. It was an example of H3 in the present identified in the Three Horizons conversation held in Fife about winter planning."

That is the value of a Three Horizons conversation. It can be started in any area, with any group, with a simple series of questions (IFF has produced a simple Kit to aid the process, but conversations can perfectly well start without it):

1. What signs do you see that the current system (or culture if you prefer this word) is under strain or even failing? (H1 strain)

2. What would an ideal system (culture) look like and how would it feel? (H3)

3. Do you know of any examples of elements of this ideal system (culture) which already exist? (H3 in the present)

4. What are the innovations already in play that are trying to change things for the better? (H2)

5. And — given the implied transition from an existing H1 to a very different H3 in previous answers — which of these innovations aim to keep H1 going (sustaining innovation) and which are nurturing qualities of H3 (transformative innovation)?

6. Next, what are the essential elements of H1 that it will be important to carry through the transition — the baby that

must not be thrown out with the bathwater? (H1 in the future.)

7. Finally, given all this, what can we now stop doing? (H1 decommissioning)

The Three Horizons conversation, which can of course be supplemented with interviews, research, data and so on, provides an initial, shared view of the territory in advance of committing to action. Ordinarily we tend to think in binary terms: the current system or an innovation, change or die. It tends to be adversarial. The introduction of a third perspective — H3 — deepens the conversation. Innovation yes — but to what end, for what purpose? Innovation in H1 tends to be instrumental: what works? But innovation with a third horizon vision in mind is much more values-based, proving that another world is possible by embodying it in the present. It is driven by belief and personal commitment.

Configure around commitment

This then is the next phase, having scanned the landscape and determined a set of aspirations and a sense of direction: declare a commitment. In the Shine story the motivating commitment was "to help older people thrive, not just survive, in their own homes". It was that commitment, rather than any set of targets, performance measures, job descriptions or partnership agreements, that became the point of stability around which the complex whirl of messy reality configured itself for the purposes of the project.

Commitment and belief are personal qualities. Expressing the project in these terms invites people to step out of their professional role and into themselves. That gives access to capacities and resources we usually keep in the background in our professional lives – our own passions and aspirations for example. Yet having the chance to express ourselves in our work turns out

to be inspiring and attractive to others who come to know or hear about it. That is partly because this kind of project explicitly acknowledges the cultural unease I have talked about elsewhere in this book and is not just another 'patch' on the system.

The commitment thus acts as an attractor for talent, enthusiasm and other resources and as a compass bearing for the purposes of navigation. Understanding the commitment in its three horizons context reveals also its roots in a shift in values and an explicit desire to change the dominant culture by doing something counter-cultural. A simple target — 'save £500,000', for example, or 'close a continuing care ward' — carries none of this power. A commitment is about ends *and* means. A commitment to shift a culture is also always about starting at a small scale: big enough to make a difference, but not so large that it will be actively suppressed by the dominant culture. The Shine story is a perfect example of this pattern: a big claim (large savings through closing a ward) based on a simple counter-cultural intervention (having a different kind of conversation) and with almost negligible — and therefore non-threatening — initial results (five people at the end of year one).

IFF has written extensively elsewhere about how to go about configuring resources around a commitment in order to get things done — notably in the chapter on 'organising' in an extensive study of the 21st century competencies, *Dancing at the Edge*[75]. It turns out we can learn a lot from the producer figure in the world of the arts — someone who marshals resources around a creative idea to make it happen. The producer does not make the art, but creates the conditions in which it can be made. The role is very different from that of the project manager, much more fluid, human, emergent, inspiring. But it is still just a role, a set of skills and behaviours, and it can be learned. The Shine project was fortunate both to understand the need for the producer competencies and to find an individual ready to step into that role. She was able to take on the learning necessary, including carrying her excellent project management expertise more lightly in order to make room for the new approach.

As the project — and the new way of working that it embodies — grows beyond the initial team so a new pattern of working begins to take shape, embracing all those involved. In the Shine project that included people from public health, community health, occupational therapy, local government, the regulators, community volunteers, social enterprises and so on. This is not an organisation, but it is organised and involves a growing number of people united around a common purpose, a set of values and a certain culture of working. Management theorists might call it an 'adhocracy', long acknowledged as one of the most creative organisational forms but — as the name suggests — usually set up on a temporary basis in order to achieve a short-term goal. IFF talks rather of an 'integrity' — equally loose and creative, but designed to maintain a moral purpose over time.

Thinking in terms of these new organisational forms provides reassurance: in breaking new ground it always helps to have a map. At least for the project leaders, understanding Shine in this way made it easier to understand how a commitment can configure a way of working. These models also invite different questions and encourage different conversations about how to scale the work without losing its integrity and suggest what needs to be deepened in the project first before it broadens its reach. In other words, once we acknowledge complexity as the context and stop trying artificially to tame or simplify it, there are tried and tested ways of operating that will deliver the results we seek.

Grow the new in the presence of the old

The Three Horizons framework naturally frames endeavours to change the system as elements in a new patterning of activity (what becomes the new business as usual) which emerges over time. In other words it encourages us to think in terms of a transition from one system or culture to another. The process

starts by planting seeds of the new culture in the soil of the old and then nurturing them to scale, connecting with other similarly inspired ventures in what is initially likely to be an unreceptive context. It takes time — usually years, perhaps decades.

This is a process of cultural leadership. Again, much has been written elsewhere about the detail of how it can be accomplished in practice[76]. Particularly appropriate for the healthcare setting is the suggestion that practitioners of this kind of innovation need to pay attention to three things: tact, timing and titration.

Tact is a reference to how we relate to the dominant systems and culture. Too many change processes demonise resistance and the old ways, writing off the 'dinosaurs' and generally getting people's backs up by making them feel wrong. When we pay more attention to the fact that the systems we are dealing with are human systems, we learn to be more tactful. We appreciate the basic systems premise that 'structure drives behaviour' and recognise that most professionals are making the best of a bad job in increasingly dysfunctional circumstances. Those professionals also have an inkling that there must be a better way and would love to give it a try, or at least provide support or cover for those who are. With tact it is possible to engage that 'third horizon' yearning in everyone, and also to work with resistance and opposition as positive sources of energy in the system.

Timing is about picking the right moment. This is patient work, conceived as part of a transition that may take a decade or more. Yet every so often an opportunity will occur for this kind of work to get a hearing at the heart of the first horizon, business as usual, structures. It might be a crisis or a critical incident or a new innovation fund or a change in key personnel. Part of the skill of the producer figure is to sense when such opportunities occur and to be constantly scanning what is sometimes called "the adjacent possible" of other opportunities to spread the culture.

Titration is about dosage. When the moment of opportunity occurs it is important not to push too far too fast, not to press for more change than the system can bear.

These three orientations of the new towards the old are critical when thinking in terms of a transition over time. It is like redesigning the plane whilst flying it: we cannot afford for the plane that is the NHS to fall out of the air, nor can we ground it for six months while we design another. We must grow the new in the presence of the old — and ultimately free up the resources sunk into the old structures and cultural frames so that they can feed the alternative. If the new and the old become too disconnected, antagonistic even, that transfer of resources is very unlikely to occur. Without a conscious effort to achieve this transition intentionally, disruptive, disjointed and desperate change is likely. In this scenario, critical collapse of the existing system ensues, followed by the slow construction of a new system only out of the wreckage of the old.

The alternative is for small groups of committed individuals to maintain a sense of purpose over time. In the face of the challenges facing today's healthcare systems I have argued that this purpose must be not simply to innovate within the healthcare system but to innovate the system itself, all the way down to its basic assumptions. Given time and space to grow, this kind of innovation will save money, improve health and increase satisfaction for the staff involved. A point will come in all such projects where the first horizon systems start to take an interest in their success and aim to 'roll out' or 'mainstream' the results.

It is at this point that the commitment to purpose may be most strongly tested. If we are ever going to succeed in shifting the culture then we must work to be followed by, rather than swallowed by, the mainstream system. The overwhelming instinct of a system in decline is to search around for innovations that will save it. But propping up the old system will not hasten the arrival of the new – and may make its eventual appearance all the more costly and painful. The ultimate aim is to transform the culture – to free up resources sunk in maintaining today's system to flow into growing a system fit for tomorrow. Hence the next stage of the Shine project involves working with the bigger organisational structures of which it is a part to encourage them to flex their first-horizon processes to make more room for radical, responsible innovation.

Finally we need to pay attention to ourselves. This can be hard and challenging work. Changing our practice means changing ourselves, and that is never easy. Instigating change that is counter-cultural means that we can feel we are swimming upstream in our organisations — which can feel exhausting and isolating. The essence of this work is personal commitment. When there is more of ourselves in the work the rewards are thrilling, but the setbacks and disappointments are also felt more deeply.

That is why in this work we need to pay particular attention to the health of the staff taking on the challenge of innovation. The means and ends are inseparable. If this is an attempt to demonstrate that another culture is possible then it needs to be authentic — not advocating for others something that staff will not take on for themselves. This was recognised in the Shine project at an early stage with the establishment of simple peer support groups — enabling amongst staff the same kinds of 'grown-up', honest, meaningful conversation that they were trying to have with their patients. Paying attention to the health of the core integrity has been seen as critical from the start. It is both a necessary investment in the long haul, and a marker of the culture that the project is trying to bring about more widely.

Alongside the producer role, these projects — indeed, I would argue, all organisations — also need a 'shepherd'. Someone needs to look after the flock, keeping a close eye on everyone in case anyone gets caught in a fence. This is a good metaphor because not everyone needs help and those who do may only need it for a short time. But without emotional and spiritual (in a non-religious sense) support, people can despair. Kitbag is one example of a resource that has been designed to support this and is being used by NHS staff in a variety of settings. Shifting the culture of healthcare so that it can again fulfil our deeper intentions is invigorating and fulfilling. But it will also demand a lot from us. It can start to ask too much. We must look after ourselves and each other. The catalyst has failed if it burns up in the experiment.

Reflection

With skill and empathy it is possible to make the transition from existing healthcare systems to a radically different configuration in the future. Everybody has a part to play. Politicians can tell the story of the transition we need to make. Finance directors and senior managers can help to keep the existing plane in the air whilst also providing space, support and encouragement to clinicians and middle managers to redesign through cultural innovation.

New forms of organisation will support this innovation in partnership with the public and people working for a common future. Everyone can be brought together around a common vision, a shared set of values and a commitment to ensure that the means are as valuable as the ends. This is humanism in action, not change driven through ideology. It can now be supported by theory and practice which embraces the complexity of the current healthcare challenge as the starting point for change.

Human beings have found ways to respond to the greatest challenges of their times not by treating them as the problems of the past, but by discovering new resources — in themselves and in their environment. This is not an easy journey. The lessons can be challenging to deep assumptions about personal and professional

identity. But the prize is great: to restore effectiveness in a healthcare system that remains accessible to all, free at the point of delivery, meeting contemporary patterns of illness and as part of an integrated approach that sustains healthy, fulfilled lives. And all that at a fraction of the current cost. The good news is — the transition has already started. I hope readers of this book will want to join me in making it a reality.

END NOTES

1. Armstrong, D. (1983) *The Politcal Anatomy of the Body: medical knowledge in the twentieth century*. Cambridge University Press.

2. Romanyshan, RD. (2001) *Mirror and Metaphor: Images and Stories of Psychological Life*. Trivium Publications.

3. Foucault, M. (1973) (English) *The Birth of the Clinic. An Archaeology of Medical Perception*. Pantheon.

4. Menzies, I. (1989) *The Functioning of Social systems as a defence against anxiety.* The Tavistock Institute of Human Relations.

5. McCluggage, WG., Walsh, MY., Thornton, CM., Hamilton, PW., Date, A., Caughley, LM., Bharucha H. 'Inter- and intra-observer variation in the histopathological reporting of cervical squamous intraepithelial lesions using a modified Bethesda grading system.' *British Journal of Obstetrics and Gynaecology* 1998; Feb;105(2):206-10.

6. Davis, D. (2007) *The Secret History of the War on Cancer*. Basic Books.

7. Poli, R. 'A note on the difference between complicated and complex social systems.' *Cadmus* 2013; 2(1): 142-147

8. Meadows, Donella. *Dancing with Systems*. Available via http://www.donellameadows.org/archives/dancing-with-systems/

9. Diabetes UK. *State of the Nation 2012 England*.

10. UK Government. Foresight Report 2007 *Tackling Obesities — Future Choices*.

11. UK Government Equalities Office (2010) *An anatomy of economic inequality in the UK*. Report of the National Equality Panel.

12. Wilkinson, R. and Pickett, K. (2009) *The Spirit Level: why more equal societies almost always do bette*r. Penguin.

13. Marmot, M. (2004) *The Status Syndrome: How Social Standing Affects Our Health and Longevity*. Holt Paperbacks.

14. BBC news report, 12 April 2010. *NHS chiefs' pay rises "double those of nurses"*.

15. Tudor Hart, J. 'The Inverse Care Law.' *The Lancet* 1970; 297: 405–412

16. Center for the Evaluative Clinical Sciences. 2007. *Supply Sensitive Care: A Dartmouth Atlas Project Brief*.

17. Suicides in the United Kingdom. 2012 Registrations. Office of National Statistics, February 2014.

18. Kentikelenis, A., Karanikolos, M,. Reeves, A., McKee, M., Stuckler, D. 'Greece Health Crisis: from austerity to denialism'. *The Lancet* 2014; 383: 748-53.

19. Kondilis, E., Giannakopoulos, S., Gavana, M., Ierodiakonou, I., Waitzkin, H., Benos, A. 'Economic Crisis, Restrictive Policies, and the Population's Health and Health Care: The Greek Case.' *American Journal of Public Health* 2013; 103(6): 973-979.

20. Parker-Pope, T. 'Suicide Rates Rise Sharply in U.S.' *New York Times* May 2 2013.

21. National Treatment Agency for Substance Misuse. *Drug Treatment 2012: progress made, challenges ahead*.

22. Department of Health. (2008) *Reducing Alcohol Harm: Health Services in England for Alcohol Misuse*. Report by the Comptroller and Auditor General.

23. Health and Social Care Information Centre. *Statistics on Alcohol: England 2012*, accessed April 29 2013.

24. Felitti, VJ., Anda, RF., Nordenberg, D., Williamson, DF., Spitz, AM., Edwards, V., Koss, MP., Marks, JS. 'Relationship of childhood abuse and household dysfunction to many of the leading causes of death in adults.' The Adverse Childhood Experiences (ACE) Study. *American Journal of Preventive Medicine* 1998, May;14(4):245-58.

25. Putnam, R. (2000) *Bowling Alone. The collapse and revival of American community*. Simon and Schuster.

26. Baumann, Z. (2003) *Liquid Lives*. Polity Press.

27. Hanlon, P. and Carlisle S. (2012) *Afternow: what next for a healthy Scotland?* Argyll Publishing.

28. Patel, R. (2007) *Stuffed and Starved: markets, power and the hidden battle for the world food system*. Portobello.

29. UK Government. Foresight 2007. *Tackling Obesities — Future Choices*.

30. Alexander, B. (2008) *The Globalisation of Addiction: a study in the poverty of spirit*. Oxford University Press.

31. Eckersley, R. 'Is modern Western culture a health hazard?' *International Journal of Epidemiology*. 2006; 35: 252-8

32. MacShane, M., in: 'NHS could be 'overwhelmed' by people with longterm conditions.' Campbell D. *The Guardian*. January 3 2014.

33. Crown Office. (2010) *An Anatomy of Economic Inequality in the UK: Report of the National Equality Panel*.

34. *Chasing Progress: beyond measuring economic growth*. New Economics Foundation. 2004.

35. Ehrenreich, B. (1971) *The American Health Empire: Power, Profit and Politics. A report from the Policy Advisory Center*. Vintage Books.

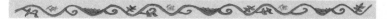

36. Figures obtained from Scottish Public Health Observatory. Incidence is derived from hospital data, mortality from the General Registrar's Office and prevalence from the Scottish Health Survey.

37. Arie, S. 'Twin Dilemma.' *British Medical Journal* 2013; 348: f7603

38. Health and Social Care Information Centre. (2012) *Prescriptions dispensed in the community: England, statistics for 2001 to 2011.*

39. Pirmohamed, M., Meakin, S., Green, C., Scott, AK., Farrar, K., Park, BK., Breckridge, AM. 'Adverse drug reactions as cause of admission to hospital: prospective analysis of 18 820 patients.' *British Medical Journal* 2004;329:15

40. Gilbert Welch, H. and Black, WC. ' Overdiagnosis in Cancer.' *Journal of the National Cancer Institute* 2010; 102(9): 605-13.

41. Jorgensen, KJ. and Gotzsche, PC. 'Overdiagnosis in publicly organised mammography screening programmes: systematic review of incidence trends.' *British Medical Journal* 2009;339:b2587

42. Moynihan, R., Doust, J., Henry, D. 'Preventing overdiagnosis: how to stop harming the healthy.' *British Medical Journal* 2012;344:e3502

43. McCartney, M. (2012) *The Patient Paradox: why sexed up medicine is bad for your health.* Pinter and Martin.

44. Heath, I. 'Overdiagnosis: when good intentions meet vested interests.' *British Medical Journal* 2013;347:f6361

45. BBC news report, 17 October 2013 . *Dorset Hospital Trusts merger plan blocked.*

46. NHS Trust Development Authority. (2013) *Securing sustainable healthcare for the people of South East London.*

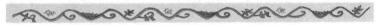

47. McMichael, AJ. 'Prisoners of the proximate: loosening the constraints on epidemiology in an age of change.' *American Journal of Epidemiology*. 1999; 149(10): 887-897

48. Cohen, D. 'FDA official: "Clinical trial system is broken".' *British Medical Journal* 2013;347:f6980

49. Goldacre, B. (2013) *Bad Pharma*. Fourth Estate.

50. Jencks, C. and Heathcote, E. (2010) *The Architecture of Hope: Maggie's Cancer Caring Centres*. Francis Lincoln.

51. Quote from Innes Pearse in Stallibrass, A. (1989) *Being Me and Also Us: lessons from the Peckham Experiment*. Scottish Academic Press.

52. Scottish Recovery Network. (2006) *Journeys of Recovery. Stories of hope and recovery from long term mental health problems*.

53. Hannah, M. and Linyard, A. 'One size fits One. Identifying and Addressing Personal Outcomes for Older People.' Health Foundation Shine 2011 Poster Presentation. Available via http://www.health.org.uk/areas-of-work/programmes/shine-eleven/related-projects/nhs-fife/learning/

54. Age UK Cornwall and Scilly (2004) *People, Place, Purpose: Shaping services around people and communities through the Newquay Pathfinder*.

55. Jaques, Elliott. (2002) *The Life and Behaviour of Living Organisms: a general theory*. Praeger.

56. Glasgow Centre for Integrative Care. Annual Report January 2013. Reilly, D. *The Healing Shift Enquiry creating a shift in health care*.

57. Pollan, M. (2008) *In Defense of Food: An Eater's Manifesto*. Penguin Group US.

58. Ornish, D. (2001) *Love and Survival: how good relationships can bring you health and well-being*. Vermillion.

59. Crisp, N. (2010) *Turning the World Upside Down: the search for global health in the 21st century*. CRC Press.

60. Moore, A., Derry, S., Eccleston, C., Kalso, E. 'Expect analgesic failure; pursue analgesic success.' *British Medical Journal* 2013; 346: f2690

61. Betsi Cadwaladar University Health Board. 'Implementation of a virtual cardiology clinic.' One of Health Foundation Shine 2010 Projects. Details available via http://www.health.org.uk/areas-of-work/programmes/ shine-ten/related-projects/betsi-cadwaladr-university/

62. Aulton, J., Ramsell, P., Kalnina, R. 'Bolton Alcohol Relapse Prevention Project.' Health Foundation Shine 2011 Poster Presentation. Available via http://www.health.org.uk/areas-of-work/programmes/shine-eleven/library/

63. Vijayaraghavan, S., Morris, J., O'Shea, T., Partlett, T., Pate, IS., Gill, M. 'DAWN: Diabetes Appointments through Webcam in Newham.' Health Foundation Shine 2011 Poster Presentation. Available via http://www.health.org.uk/areas-of-work/programmes/shine-eleven/library/

64. Mowat, H., Bunniss, S., Kelly, E. 'Community Chaplaincy Listening: Working with General Practitioners to support patient wellbeing.' *The Scottish Journal of Healthcare Chaplaincy*, 2012; Vol 15 (1): 21-26

65. Ballatt, J., Campling, P. (2011) *Intelligent Kindess*. Royal College Psychotherapy Publications.

66. Hannah, M. and McNidder R.(2013) *Using Kitbag to support staff in mental health teams*. Health and Social Care Chaplaincy. 2013; Vol 1 (1): 61-66

67. Frankl, Victor. (2004) *Man's Search for Meaning*. (First published in English in 1959) Random House.

68. Murray, K. 'How Doctors Choose to Die.' *The Guardian* 8 February 2012. Available via http://www.theguardian.com/society/2012/feb/08/how-doctors-choose-die

69. Health and Social Care Information Centre. *Sickness absence rates in the NHS January to March 2013*. http://www.hscic.gov.uk/catalogue/PUB11194

70. Campbell, D. 'Growing exodus of A&E doctors to Australia adds to strain on NHS.' *The Guardian* 27 December 2013. http://www.theguardian.com/society/2013/dec/27/exodus-nhs-doctors-australia

71. Crisp, N. (2010) *Turning the World Upside Down: the search for global health in the 21st Century*. Royal Society of Medicine Press.

72. See for example: Warner, N., O'Sullivan, J. (2014) *Solving the NHS Cash and Care crisis: routes to health and care renewal*. Reform.
Appleby, J., Galea, A., Murray, R. (2014) *The NHS Productivity Challenge: Experience from the front line*. Kings Fund.
Roberts, A., Marshal, IL., Charlesworth, A. (2012) *A decade of austerity? The funding pressures facing the NHS 2011/13 to 2021/22*. Nuffield Trust.

73. See for example: Yudkin, JS., Montori, VM. 'The epidemic of pre-diabetes: the medicine and the politics.' *British Medical Journal*. 2014;349:g4485
Glasziou, P., Moynihan, R., Richards, T., Godlee, F. 'Too much medicine; too little care.' *British Medical Journal* 2013;347:f4247
Moynihan, R. 'Science of overdiagnosis to be served up with a dose of humility.' *British Medical Journal* 2013;347:f5157

74. Sharpe, B. (2013) *Three Horizons: The Patterning of Hope*. Triarchy Press.

75. O'Hara, M., Leicester, G. (2013) *Dancing at the Edge: Competence, culture and organisation in the 21st century.* Triarchy Press.

76. See for example: Leicester, G. 'Transformative Innovation and the Policymaker of the Future', in *ETHOS* Issue 13 June 2014, Civil Service College Singapore; or Leicester G, 'Real Cultural Leadership: leading the culture in a time of cultural crisis', in *A Cultural Leadership Reader* edited by Sue Kay and Katie Venner with Susanne Burns and Mary Schwarz, Arts Council England (2010)

About the Author

Margaret Hannah is a Consultant in Public Health Medicine and has worked in the NHS for over twenty years. She is currently Deputy Director of Public Health in NHS Fife and Honorary Senior Lecturer at St Andrews University.

A member of International Futures Forum for many years, she has developed IFF Kitbag – a set of resources to promote psychological capacity in times of radical change. This book represents a personal and IFF view, not that of her employer.

About the Illustrator

JENNIFER Williams is critically acclaimed at making hand-made books, cut outs, photographs, illustrations, prints and puppets.

She is a trustee and member of International Futures Forum and for 31 years directed the Centre for Creative Communities.

International Futures Forum

INTERNATIONAL Futures Forum (IFF) is a non-profit organisation established to support a transformative response to complex and confounding challenges and to restore the capacity for effective action in today's powerful times.

At the heart of IFF is a deeply informed inter-disciplinary and international network of individuals from a range of backgrounds covering a wide range of diverse perspectives, countries and disciplines. The group meets as a learning community as often as possible, including in plenary session. And it seeks to apply its learning in practice. IFF takes on complex, messy, seemingly intractable issues - notably in the arenas of health, learning, governance and enterprise - where paradox, ambiguity and complexity characterise the landscape, where rapid change means yesterday's solution no longer works, where long-term needs require a long-term logic and where only genuine innovation has any chance of success.
www.internationalfuturesforum.com

Triarchy Press

TRIARCHY Press is an independent publisher of new alternative thinking (altThink) about organisations and society, and practical ways to apply that thinking. In our partnership with IFF we are lucky to work with some of the most inspiring thinkers and practitioners in the field. They challenge us to embrace the potential of change rather than retreat into the familiar – revealing wiser ways of preparing for an uncertain future.

Other IFF titles include: *Three Horizons, Dancing at the Edge, Ten Things to do in a Conceptual Emergency, Ready for Anything, Economies of Life, Beyond Survival: A Short Course in Pioneering* and *Transformative Innovation in Education (2nd Edition)*.
www.triarchypress.net.

Printed in September 2019
by Rotomail Italia S.p.A., Vignate (MI) - Italy